Let Me Turn You On

LET ME TURN YOU ON

The Secrets to Activating Your
Deep Core Muscles

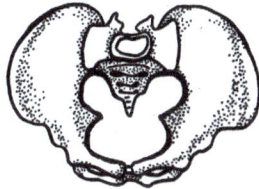

Jeanie Iverson Crawford,
DPT, CAPP-PELVIS, CMTPT, BIKEPT

Disclaimer: The information and opinions contained in this book are for educational purposes only. The information does not consider any particular person's specific medical condition. The information and opinions expressed should not be construed as medical advice or an exact treatment plan for any particular condition. You should always consult with your medical doctor before starting, stopping, or changing any specific health care treatment and/or prescription.

First Edition 2025.

Cover art designed by Jeanie Iverson Crawford, illustrated by Renee Zupancich.

ISBN 979-8-218-73892-1

This book is dedicated to
William Iverson Crawford

CONTENTS

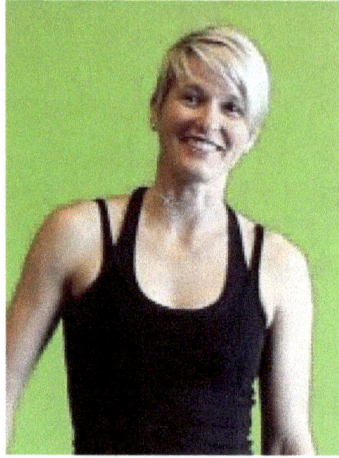

The Author

PREFACE

WHO AM I AND WHAT DO I HAVE TO SAY!

After receiving an undergraduate degree in Kinesiology from the University of Minnesota, I graduated from Slippery Rock University of Pennsylvania with a Doctorate in Physical Therapy. But my education didn't stop there; I have devoted a great deal of time going above and beyond state requirements with continuing education. I have certification in the area of the pelvis through the American Physical Therapy Association and I hold an additional certification in manual trigger point therapy. I have over twenty years of clinical practice in the area of the pelvis.

I have practiced in multiple specialties, including vestibular, pelvis, spinal, sports injuries, pre- and post-surgeries, falls and balance, and men's and women's health. I have traveled to many states and worked in many settings, giving me broad insight into a plethora of approaches for diagnosing and treating problematic areas with physical therapy.

As a proud and adventurous mother of two boys, I relate to and enjoy restoring the athleticism of mothers, which is sadly often lost postpartum. I currently practice as a Doctor of Physical Therapy in a small historical city in Wisconsin. As owner and founder of SBR Therapy and Wellness Clinic, I focus on Swim Bike Run athletes and their ailments. I am on a "damn good mission" to create a place for athletes and inspiring athletes to find answers to the ailments affecting their sports performance or their ability to participate in physical activity, a place for true, long-lasting results for life and sport. I prefer to call myself a bodyworker, using my experienced hands and intention to manipulate or assist the body in restoring homeostasis.

I would like to thank the the many experiences in life that I've been fortunate to have. These experiences have allowed me to better learn and study the body from many angles. Thanks to my ancestors and creators. Thanks to my parents and siblings for making smart choices and allowing a relatively financially and emotionally stress free upbringing. My nuclear unit — thank you! Thank you to my husband, Danny, who allowed numerous continuing education courses and late nights writing and studying, as well as time to just breathe and think and work out. Thank you to all who have accepted my out-of-box learning and enhanced it. Thank you to my unofficial-official editor, Mary Catherine Jones, who assisted me in my writing, and my official editor Gabriel.

Jeanie Iverson Crawford,
DPT, CAPP-PELVIS, CMTPT, BIKEPT

INTRODUCTION

Just as a flower or tree thrives when it is correctly cared for, I can promise that you will feel a faster and more sustainable improvement in your well-being when you optimize your deep core. These are the results that my patients and I have had by using my techniques. Scientifically and logically, it all makes sense. So let me show you how to thrive!

In this book, you will hear some of my mind. I will share multiple clinical insights and thoughts that will assist you in looking outside the box, or deeper inside the box. I try to provide logical information to treat and prevent ailments and enhance performance. I'm providing this information in a very straightforward and concise manner. I describe the mechanics, proper care, and maintenance of the body. Emphasis is on the importance of your own senses and how they can be used to discover essential deep core muscles that once *turned on* will provide a solid frame for both physical and personal satisfaction. Let me show you how to get *turned on* and prevent needless pain, suffering, and unnecessary surgeries and medical bills. Let me save you and your family some money!

WHO WILL BENEFIT FROM THIS BOOK?

The General Public and Athletes

Almost everyone has some issue or another with alignment, or strength, or pain, or stability, or breathing, or sex, or circulation, etc.

This book can help with these issues. People wanting to change their image from the inside out will find many tips and exercises. Athletes looking to gain an edge in competition will also benefit from the techniques described here in detail.

Health Care Professionals

Physical therapists, biomechanics, chiropractors, massage therapists, doctors and nurses, athletic and personal trainers...

Parents and Schoolteachers

Parents and schoolteachers can get a jump-start on encouraging the health of their children or students by understanding core mechanics and implementing exercises to strengthen the core.

Certain Patient Populations
or Individuals with Particular Diagnoses

- Pregnancy, or history of pregnancy
- Spine issues, including chronic pain, scoliosis, or musculoskeletal imbalance
- Lung issues, including chronic obstructive pulmonary disease, cystic fibrosis, or asthma
- Sexual issues, including decreased libido, pain, or sexual dysfunction
- Gastrointestinal issues, including gastroesophageal reflux disease (GERD) or constipation

- Incontinence of the bladder and/or bowel
- Orthopedic diagnoses, including pain in joints, muscles, or tendons

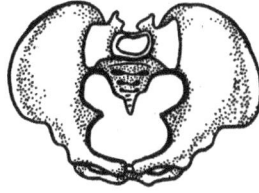

GETTING *TURNED ON*

I became interested in the specialized niche of women's health within physical therapy when I was seventeen years old. While enrolled as a kinesiology student at the University of Minnesota, I started volunteering at the nearby Institute of Athletic Medicine. I remember being very excited to shadow the women's health specialists. Given that I was shadowing *women's* specialists at an *athletic* medicine institute, I thought I would be working primarily with female athletes. To my surprise, most of the patients that we saw were not actually athletes. Certainly any athlete would benefit from seeing an integrative and dynamic pelvic floor therapist to enhance their performance. Although I firmly believe that everyone has an inner athlete lurking inside them, my experience at the time did not involve the patient population or the type of therapy I had imagined.

I soon learned that women's health specialists worked with patients of all ages, women and men, if they had problems involving the pelvis. Some of these problems or diagnoses included incontinence, postpartum issues, erectile dysfunction, dyspareunia (pain during intercourse), prolapse (where internal body parts descend or begin to exit through the vagina or rectum), pelvic pain (including strains or sprains of the abductor muscles and abdominal or groin pain), and many other types of pelvic discomfort. Although it was not what I expected, my experience at the Institute of Athletic Medicine lit a spark; it was to be the first of many experiences that I undertook to gain insight into the deep core.

I continued to be interested in working in women's health while studying physical therapy in graduate school. And I studied women's health issues and treatments while taking multiple jobs throughout the United States after becoming licensed. After securing a position with an outpatient rehabilitation and "sport" medicine clinic, more than fifty percent of my caseload over the course of ten years was for pelvic floor issues.

The point is, during that time, the more patients I saw and treated hands-on, the more I learned about how essential the correct functioning of the deep core muscles was to overall health. This specific muscle group was very special, very powerful, and quite vital for multiple reasons that went well beyond pelvic issues. Many times, working on the core would alleviate multiple types of musculoskeletal pain and biomechanical ailments, including common musculoskeletal problems such as low back pain, plantar fasciitis, patellofemoral syndrome, and sprains and strains of the groin or hamstrings. Strengthening and restoring the deep core also helped with medical diagnoses such as acid reflux, digestion issues (such as irritable bowel syndrome or constipation), speaking, etc.

Although activating these muscles is not my only source of success with my patients, it is an essential part, and the primary topic I will discuss in this book. My goal is to treat the greater community, to do good, to make people feel a sense of deep health inside their body, which is, in my opinion, a temple for their spirit to move in on this earth.

THE KEY TO THE CORE: THE PELVIS

Focusing on the deep muscles of the pelvis directed me to examine wholeness throughout the entire body. I truly believe that the pelvis is the key connection within the whole body. The desired state of wholeness is necessary to enable the upper body to function smoothly along with the whole lower body. When repairing a body, if I had to choose one place to begin, I would start by making sure that the pelvis is aligned and the associated muscles are working with normal biomechanics. An experienced pelvic physical therapist will tell you that in order to repair and strengthen the pelvis, you will often *not* start by directly treating the pelvic floor. I do believe that it is helpful, and, in many situations, necessary to identify, isolate, and strengthen the pelvic floor at some point during the recovery of the pelvis in order to achieve normal alignment, mobility, strength, and function. But the goal is that the foundation is corrected.

As a pelvic floor physical therapist, I have done a lot of work internally — both rectally and vaginally — while working on the pelvic floor muscles. This forces me to *feel* instead of see to assess and treat. Therefore, I have learned to *think* a little differently. As I have had to explore these muscles with touch and listening instead of sight, I have found that I receive more accurate, informative, and educational feedback about how the body really works. In fact, I do a lot of my work with my eyes closed. At times I even analyze running and walking form with my eyes closed, just listening and feeling. Interestingly, while I was assessing one of my patients who is a caregiver with my eyes closed, she said that her blind patient had told her she was walking with a limp. Yes, the legally blind can see so much more. Be aware that people who are blind may see you more clearly than many other people will ever see you — they have identified me by both sound and smell. The goal is for my readers to see the deep core more clearly, and often we have to do this *without* our eyesight.

Many times, I have asked my patients what the most beneficial part of their pelvic floor therapy has been. They usually respond that as much as they may not like it, the manual pelvic floor therapy, consisting of manual internal vaginal and rectal work, seems to offer the most benefit. I believe that this is because the patients are now also challenged to think differently; they are forced to identify their body from a state of feeling and listening instead of sight. They are given a new path to insight into their own body and healing.

Patients have also added that follow-up education gives them a sense of reassurance about the therapy they have undertaken and allows them to consider whether newfound function seems normal or abnormal to them. Having a conversation, with feedback given and received in both directions, is very helpful in both formulating a treatment plan and allowing the patient to feel confident about the choices that they are making for their body. Often patients are worried and do not know what is making their body worse or better. They do not know what normal is or how to get there. Education on normal mechanics and what patients should or should not do is inspirational and allows patients to move forward with confidence.

So often the medical field has us living in fear. For example, they will say, "don't do that if it hurts." Sometimes this is true, oftentimes it is not. We cannot always move forward and make progress by completely avoiding pain. We need to investigate the cause of the pain and work towards fixing it. A diagnosis is often blamed as the cause of all of a patient's pain, and again, this is often not the case. To gain true body insight, it is essential to see a qualified therapist. We physical therapists are the musculoskeletal doctors. But note that just like any group of professionals, we are not all the same. For example, we all function at different levels and with different expertise. Therefore, if you don't find your answers with one therapist, find another who is more qualified for your needs and wants.

WHAT MAKES THE DEEP CORE MUSCLES SO DIFFERENT?

Why are these muscles so underappreciated and rarely looked at? Unlike other muscles in the body, the deep core muscles are not easily visible since they are buried deep inside of you. As a result, they often receive little or no attention.

In contrast, most people can identify the location of their biceps, rectus abdominis (commonly referred to as the "six-pack"), quadriceps, etc. You can easily see the bicep lengthen and shorten when you are doing something as simple as lifting a glass of milk. These particular muscles are surface-visible and easy to identify. It is certainly understandable why there is an immediate sense of satisfaction in seeing visible muscles such as the biceps or quadriceps become strengthened, toned, and enlarged.

The deep muscles, on the other hand, are not so obvious at first. Their importance is overshadowed by the visible muscles such as those previously mentioned. Once you learn to identify the deep muscles, however, they become more important in your overall view of body strength. They become very clear and very sexy. The deep core muscles provide significant body stability, strength, and mobility. Furthermore, if you are breathing correctly, they are always coiling and recoiling — contracting and relaxing — and functioning with your every breath. They assist in keeping you alive.

The problem that arises is that because the deep core muscles are harder to see, they can be harder to actually *turn on*. One has to learn how to identify them in the mind and also how to find them, directly or indirectly, through their overlying tissues.

WHY ARE THESE DEEP CORE MUSCLES IMPORTANT?

A major job of the pelvic floor muscles and other deep core muscles of the torso (or back) is that they provide strength and stability. The deep core is *your* base of support — these muscles are your roots. The deep core is your foundation; it is what your extremities need to push and pull off of. The deep core muscles prevent you from swaying in any direction, provided they are symmetrical, mobile, and can handle resistance. The deep core is your set of roots for being grounded, stable, and providing strength to the rest of your body.

Your deep core muscles are also some of the closest muscles to your central nervous system, which is the brain and spinal cord. These muscles assist in keeping the spinal cord and brain together for communicating. Furthermore, they assist to keep the peripheral nervous system connected to the central nervous system. Nerves are our vital lines for the body to communicate with itself and the surrounding environment.

A WEAK DEEP CORE CAN AFFECT YOUR EXTREMITIES AND,
VICE VERSA, A WEAK AND/OR TIGHT EXTREMITY
CAN AFFECT YOUR DEEP CORE

One of my theories is as follows: if your deep core is strong, it does not need extensions such as the extremities (arms, legs, neck) to assist in holding it up. Often I see the extremities compensating for a weak deep core. Just as a tree with a weak base might need cables or ropes to hold it up, similarly, a weak deep core might need extremities to help hold the core or body up. This is often what I see clinically.

Your body is only as strong as your foundation. When your deep core muscles can hold you up, the extremities can then act separately from the rest of the body as they are meant to. The core is for stability and breathing. Extremities should be able to function freely from your core, and should not need to be used to hold your core up. For example, it is common to see the hip flexors being used to stabilize the lumbopelvic junction, as they connect to the front of your vertebrae.

HOW ELSE ARE DEEP CORE MUSCLES DIFFERENT?
THEY ARE ALL BREATHING MUSCLES

Not only does the deep core stabilize and allow symmetry, all of the deep core muscles assist with *breathing*. Again, when your deep core is weak, the extremities will start to act as extensions, like stakes or cables, to keep you upright. The extremities and long muscles of the spine can also start to act as breathing muscles, taking on the job of weak deep core muscles.

I found this out firsthand in class one day when I wanted to release my latissimus dorsi — the largest of the back muscles. My class partner employed a technique called *dry needling* (the insertion of a thin, acupuncture-style needle into a pressure point) to cause that muscle to release, but the muscle simply twitched fifty or more times instead of releasing. From this experience I learned that the body will always choose first to breathe — and at that time, my body was using my latissimus dorsi muscle to breathe.

Other common muscles used for breathing by people with a weak core are the pectoral muscles (chest), the scalene muscles (a group of three pairs of muscles in the neck), and the upper trapezius muscles (back). Being aware of these compensatory strategies, I have become selective when needling patients. Before I needle compensatory muscles (in this case, any muscle that is potentially doing the job of the breathing muscles) or accessory muscles (in this case, muscles used to assist with labored breathing), I make sure patients are not using them to breathe at rest. It would be a waste of time to needle compensatory muscles currently being used for breathing until I teach the patient to breathe properly.

One of my therapy techniques is to work the deep core, which in turn will assist in freeing the extremities from the core. Another one of my techniques is to release the extremities from the core so the core can function without restriction. Achieving proper core function is a careful balancing act. If, for example, your arms are "glued" down to your ribs, then your arms and ribs cannot move freely as they are meant to. Your ribs and rib muscles should be used to assist in breathing and your arms and arm muscles should be used to carry things. In order to fix this problem, I would focus on both strengthening the deep core and releasing the arm muscles and fascia from the rib cage.

STRENGTHENING THE DESIRED PATHWAY

Your body will often choose the path of least resistance when it has become programmed in either a positive or negative way. This is specifically the case when it comes to breathing. As a result, the longer your body is in a compensated neuromuscular (brain-to-body) pattern, the harder it can be to change the pattern. Your circuits (nerve pathways) become hardwired the longer you repeat motor functions, whether for good or bad. Motor functions are the tasks you do every day: walking, squatting, biking, running, etc. How you perform these motor functions will determine whether or not your body mechanics are being strengthened or weakened through movement. The brain does not always do what is right for the body. The brain does what it is taught and what it is able to do with its current restrictions. I'm mainly talking musculoskeletal, but emotions also take part in the function of the musculoskeletal and fascial system.

It is important to change any abnormalities in your body. Unless you make doable changes, you will become misaligned and weakened. The breathing muscles — your deep core — will be overtaken. This can leave you with poor body mechanics. Think about the previous example where the arm is "glued down" to the ribs. This "gluing" of the shoulder girdle to the ribs will eventually affect the normal functions of both the ribs and the shoulder/arm. Thinking even further beyond the level of the shoulder girdle and the ribs, these pulls can start to affect the entire body at levels above and below.

DEEP CORE MUSCLES ARE NOT EASILY *TURNED ON*

Unlike the long muscles of the extremities or spine, the deep core muscles are not easily turned back on when turned off. For multiple reasons, it is important that our deep core muscles are *turned on. Are you turned on? And what does this mean?*

Just like a light bulb, our muscles have the ability to turn off or turn on. Sometimes after an accident, surgery, overuse, or underuse, our deep core muscles turn off. This can happen to any muscle, but our focus here is on the deep core. Unlike other muscles, it takes some effort to turn the deep core muscles back on. Studies have shown that even years later, these muscles can remain dormant.[1] Personally and professionally, I can attest to this finding whole-heartedly.

When the deep core muscles turn off, the body adapts and compensates. Many times, you will not even notice or feel any pain. Other times, it will be very obvious.

Consider the patient who lifts something heavy and gets immediate back pain, causing them to be unable to stand up straight or walk. A couple of days later, they are back to their normal activities or daily living, saying their pain is gone. Often, the pain is gone because the affected area has shut down. The deep core, especially the multifidi muscles (see Figure 1; see chapter "Multifidi"), are often turned off with this type of back injury. The body has simply compensated so one might appear to move unharmed from one's injury.

Eventually, we run out of compensations; the patient now looks like a chronic pain patient. Many body compensations later and no longer able to bypass an area of injury, normal mechanics, after multiple mishaps, have not been restored. New pathways have been formed from the brain to the muscles to create movement. It is common to see swelling in areas where the multifidi muscles have turned off; with time this can cause a chronic ache with prolonged work, standing, or sitting. When particularly bad, the multifidi muscles are no longer able to assist with decompressing the vertebral joints and nerves, leading to constant pain.

If a muscle is not *turned on*, it is not able to complete its job and the body is forced to compensate. This compensation can lead to misalignment, poor body mechanics, and less efficiency. All of these things can make a person look and feel old. Unless trained to identify these muscles, you might not even know that the deep core is no longer working for you.

Studies have shown that the body remembers both pain and the movement associated with pain, and then learns to adapt quickly. For example, in one study by Hodges et al., patients were told to take a step down off of a low, five centimeter step.[2] The study was set up so that the second that the patient's foot hit the ground, pain was transmitted to their sacrum by the researchers. Afterwards, each time that the patient made a downward step, the hip and pelvic muscles were overly recruited (locked up in response), even when pain was not transmitted by the researchers.

The above study demonstrates how your mechanics can change quickly, and even unnecessarily, after you experience pain or injury. For example, the mechanics of your hip can be changed by simply stepping off a curb that you miscalculated to be higher or lower than it actually is. The brain remembers and creates "motor memory." When you take a step off of a curb that you did not see, or did not think was so high at the time, and then experience pain, your hip may now continue to lock up with every subsequent step to prevent pain from happening again. Not to mention that the step off of that curb could have caused misalignment at the hip and pelvis, an area that is now locked up or out of place, in addition to demonstrating poor muscle motor behaviors.

WHAT *TURNS YOU ON*?

Another interesting characteristic of the deep core muscles is that people connect with these muscles individually and differently, both to turn them on and to identify and isolate them for strengthening purposes. Because everyone connects with their deep core muscles in a different way, a set of tips to ignite them might work for one person and not for another. So how do we train these deep core muscles if everyone identifies with them differently? What turns you on might not turn someone else on. A set of verbal cues from the brain to the body is one of the keys to get these core muscles to work for you. In this book, more on cues and other ways to *turn on* the deep core will be highlighted.

THE DEEP CORE HAS THE ABILITY TO
TURN YOU AND OTHERS ON

Although these muscles are not easily seen or turned on, once they are on, an added bonus is that, yes, these muscles can help you become *turned on* and they can *turn on* others. In their state of physical action, and when they are on display, these muscles are incredibly sexy to observe. These muscles shape you. They are your framework. They are your *image*.

It is such a turn on to see someone's deep core contracting and relaxing in a state of balance. It is biomechanically attractive as a bodyworker to see a healthy machine. But many people also unconsciously feel the deep core to be hot and sexy, and rightfully so. Watch a healthy core as the ribs coil and recoil on all sides — this is POWER. A healthy core shows mobility, symmetry, and balance. The deep core is like good artwork or architectural design; we all know what looks good, but true artists understand the balance involved in the process and *really* see it. I want to show you what a healthy deep core really looks like!

Look at the bodies of consistently successful elite athletes. With each breath they take, they move their whole core from pelvis to neck. Like a healthy newborn baby, you simply have to look at them to see they are alive. This is because they are using their whole core to breathe, as we all should. But *no*, most of the population does not know or remember, or is unable to breathe normally. I know this because I instinctively study people's biomechanics daily. Plus, people tell me when I am fixing them. They will say, "I never knew about that, and I go to yoga," or "Why isn't everyone taught this?" or "I cannot expand my ribs there," or "How did I forget how to breathe?"

The deep core shapes successful athletes, allowing the long muscles of the torso and extremities to have a solid base to push and pull from. The result? They are able to improve their performance. Now, most athletes have no idea about their deep core. Most have never had a pelvic floor exam. Most have never had a "deep core training day." They simply have never lost their form, or perform specific exercises that tend to keep these deep muscles strong. Many professionals and elite athletes also get manual bodywork done, which can assist in keeping the body aligned and turned on. Many also focus heavily on form, posture, and the relaxing and contracting of specific muscles, which will assist with keeping the deep core on. And rest — elite athletes know that rest is as equally important as the training. Rest is also important to keep the deep core muscles healthy, that is, *turned on* and functioning with full range of motion and with proper biomechanics and neuromuscular patterning.

Just to be clear, though, plenty of elite athletes have weak cores that could be significantly helped. Many have had to end their careers because they never recovered from biomechanical problems that resulted in poor performance, injury, and/or too much pain.

Now, it is not enough to just have the deep core muscles on; these muscles need to be able to coil and recoil. They need to have their full mobility. One needs to learn to bring the deep core muscles from a shortened to a lengthened position and then back again. Both the *visible* and *invisible* muscles need to be *turned on* and functioning with full range of motion at their shortest and longest states. You won't always need to bring them to their full ranges, but you should train them in order to maximize their potential. You might only require these muscles to be functioning in the middle range, depending on the movements that you are performing. However, using an arm as an example, why settle for an arm that cannot fully extend or bend? You want full mobility in the arm, just as you want full mobility in the deep core.

Sometimes the core muscles are stuck in an "on" state in either a lengthened or shortened position. Again, you not only need to have these muscles *turned on*, they need to be able to coil and recoil, lengthen and shorten, correctly. Pay attention to a three-month-old child for an example of correct movement and functionality. The child's body is coiling and recoiling from neck to pelvis. The abdominals are moving, expanding and hollowing. The ribs are rising and falling on all planes. This is a constant state of blood flow and a constant state of *healthy* movement.

Try to bring the deep core muscles to their end ranges each day. Many times, you may think your muscles are at their end range of motion, only to learn that your perception is inaccurate, based on limited ranges you have been living with for years or decades. At such times, try to stretch past your perceived end ranges, especially when working with the intercostal muscles to restore full inhalation capacity (see chapter "Intercostals"). You cannot always go to your physical therapist, athletic trainer, or yoga instructor, and definitely not to your doctor; they likely do not know what normal range is, and they certainly never assess the deep core. Many doctors are adapting slowly to more holistic treatments, away from surgery and drugs. Some are attempting physical therapy approaches more often now. But most providers DO NOT SEE or KNOW HOW TO SEE or turn these muscles on. You must go to someone who specializes in the deep core and truly works on developing it.

YOUR DECOMPRESSION SYSTEM

One amazing function of your deep core is that it is a built-in decompression system. Imagine your breath as a shock absorber. Through the action of coiling and recoiling, the breath compresses and decompresses your body. For example, with every deep breath of a healthy core, you are providing natural traction on your spine. You are able to see the action of the intercostals and diaphragm expanding the ribs and indirectly decompressing the vertebra. The deep core provides natural decompression and brilliant natural traction, taking the load off with every breath, preventing wear and tear on your spinal joints.

YOUR DEEP CORE SHAPES, BALANCES, AND ALIGNS *YOU!*

When you think more about the coiling and recoiling of every breath, you realize that the breath is actually *shaping you.* What shape would you have if you could not breathe into your lungs? When *turned on,* the core muscles align the spine. A powerful core allows the long muscles of the spine and extremities to be free, which creates a different shape than long muscles that are asked to function for a weak core. Everything becomes more aligned and balanced when all of the deep muscles are on and symmetrically working.

Balance and alignment occur when the muscles are operating symmetrically on all planes — front/back, left/right, and rotationally. The coiling and recoiling of your core maintains constant blood flow and prevents stagnation in the body. You will learn more about how the deep core is working constantly to shape you as you read this book!

The purpose of this book is to *turn you on.* I want to teach you how to truly identify these deep core muscles, to really see them, to know if they are not only on, but functioning to full capacity. I want you to understand why these muscles are so vitally important for your overall health. These muscles have the capacity to affect your mind, body, and spirit — and improve your sport and life.

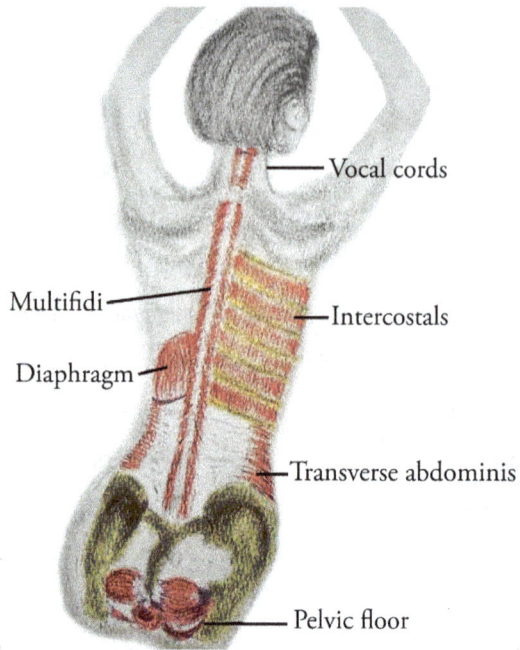

Figure 1. The deep core muscles.
Art by Renee Zupancich.

WHAT ARE THE DEEP CORE MUSCLES?

Keep in mind that some health care professionals will subtract or add other muscles into the definition of the deep core. I think most practitioners who specialize in the deep core would agree that these six are the primary muscles of the deep core (see Figure 1):

- Pelvic floor (levator ani muscles)
- Transverse abdominis
- Multifidi

- Intercostals
- Diaphragm
- Vocal cords/laryngeal muscles

WHAT DO THE DEEP CORE MUSCLES HAVE IN COMMON?

- They are difficult for the average person to see and feel.
- They are an essential part of normal breathing.
- They provide a stable foundation for the rest of the body.
- They seek symmetry on all planes — left/right, front/back, and rotationally — which assists with alignment and balance.
- Once turned off, they do not automatically turn back on with movement.
- Often, they require mental focus and imaging techniques to turn back on.

REFERENCES

1. Hides JA, Stokes MJ, Saide M, Jull GA, Cooper DH. Evidence of lumbar multifidus muscle wasting ipsilateral to symptoms in patients with acute/subacute low back pain. *Spine.* 1994;19:165-172. doi: 10.1097/00007632-199401001-00009

2. Hodges PW, Tsao H, Sims K. Gain of postural responses increases in response to real and anticipated pain. *Experimental Brain Research.* 2015;233:2745-2752. doi: 10.1007/s00221-015-4347-0

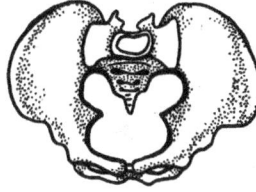

PELVIC FLOOR

In general, the pelvic floor muscles connect from the sacrum to your pubic bone like a bowl or a hammock. The pelvic floor muscles are found in what many people in earlier times described as the "sacred area." I would agree with that description. The pelvic floor is very powerful when working. When it is not, it can be disruptive to our spiritual, mental, physical, and sexual well-being. A lack of energy, strength, and mobility in this muscle group is certainly not ideal for a variety of reasons, as discussed below.

A BREAKDOWN OF THE PELVIC FLOOR MUSCLES

The pelvic floor muscles are known as the *levator ani*. The levator ani is a group of three to six muscles, depending on the book you study. The simplified list includes the pubococcygeus, the iliococcygeus, and the coccygeus, described below (see Figure 2.1). These muscles as a group help to form a bowl or U-shaped sling. The pelvic floor can also be known as the "Kegel muscle," a term coined by Dr. Kegel to describe this region and his method for using pelvic floor contractions to treat incontinence.

Pubococcygeus

The pubococcygeus is one of the pelvic floor muscles, which some divide into the puborectalis, pubovaginalis, and pubococcygeus. In essence, these muscle fibers as a group go from the pubic bone and surrounding fascia to the coccyx (the tailbone). This muscle is at the midline of the body. During a digital vaginal exam, this muscle is the most immediate and medial muscle felt at the entrance of the hiatus (opening) of the vagina.

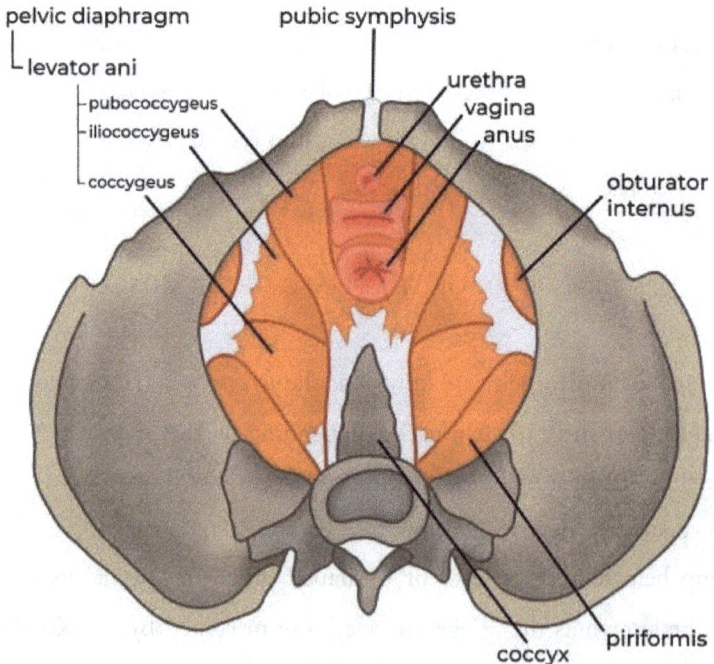

Figure 2.1. Superior view of the female pelvic diaphragm. Adapted from Jinnicha/*Shutterstock.com.*

Origin: Pubic symphysis, fascia of urogenital diaphragm (see Figure 2.2).[1]

Location/Insertion: Midline sling posterior to the rectum, coccyx, and sacrum (see Figure 2.3).[1]

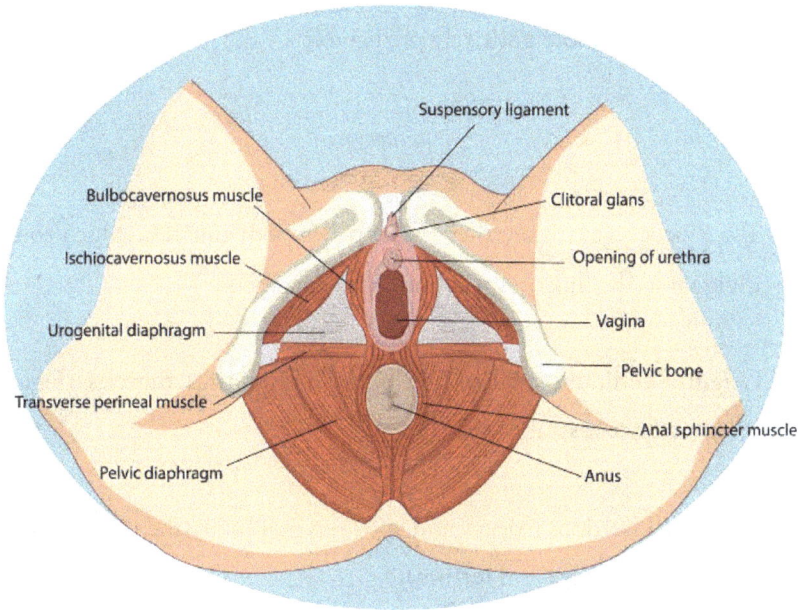

Figure 2.2. Inferior view of the female pelvis.
Adapted from Mister_X/*Shutterstock.com*.

Clinical Notes: The pubococcygeus can often be too tight in people experiencing constipation, pain with bowel movements, inability to have a bowel movement, or pain with intercourse. It is also associated with prostatitis. When this muscle is too tight, women are unable to have vaginal penetration or have only a limited amount of vaginal penetration available. This muscle is often felt to be tight with certain emotional issues, including sexual abuse, abortion, or unplanned pregnancies. Interestingly, it can be significantly tight at one internal assessment and looser at another. Meaning, I can perform manual internal work at some visits, while at other visits it is impossible to insert even a pinky finger into the vagina and/or rectum. As biomechanics and alignment improve, activation and strength of the pelvic floor becomes more positively predictable.

Iliococcygeus

The iliococcygeus is another of the pelvic floor muscles, which some divide into the iliococcygeus and ischiococcygeus.

Origin: Tendinous arch of the obturator internus muscles (Figure 2.1) and fascia, ischium.[1]

Location/Insertion: Coccyx and anococcygeal body (the fibrous tissue between the coccyx and rectum).[1]

Clinical Notes: This muscle is commonly felt as weak with patients who have incontinence and vaginal prolapse. The obturator internus muscle acts to externally rotate the hip and has a direct connection to the rim of the pelvic floor, the tendinous arch (which is a firm rim like the rim of a bowl). Because the pelvic floor attaches to the obturator internus muscle and its fascia, the obturator internus muscle can indirectly pull up on the pelvic floor when it is activated or if it is tight. This can create problems with the pelvic floor muscles, as they are constantly getting pulled on.

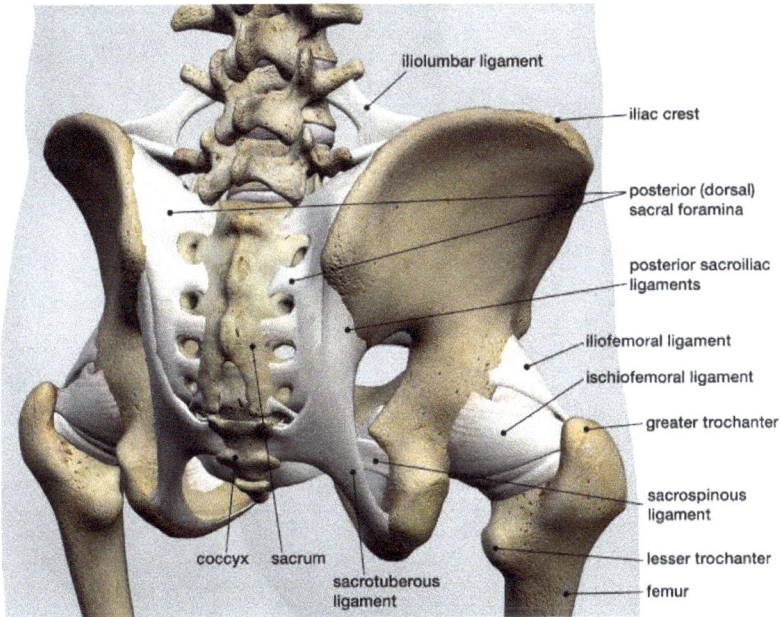

Figure 2.3. The bony and ligamentous support of the pelvis: posterior view. From Hank Grebe/*Shutterstock.com.*

Coccygeus

I consider the coccygeus to be another one of the pelvic floor muscles. However, some separate it from the other pelvic floor muscles or levator ani. It is the bulk of the muscle of the pelvic floor on the back end near the tailbone.

Origin: Sacrospinous ligament (see Figure 2.4), spine of the ischium.[1]

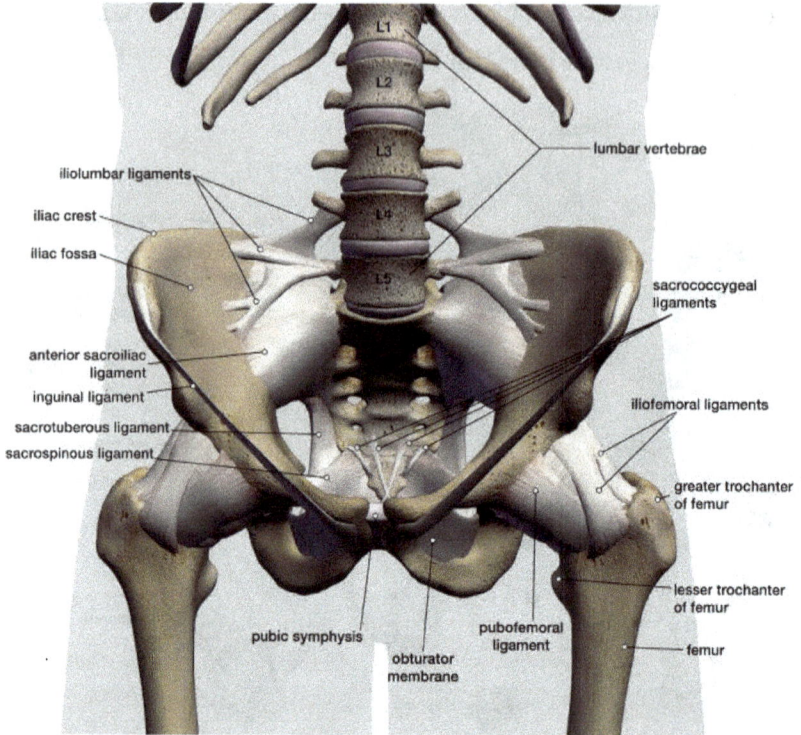

Figure 2.4. The bony and ligamentous support of the pelvis: anterior/frontal view. Adapted from Hank Grebe/*Shutterstock.com.*

Location/Insertion: Anococcygeal body and coccyx (tailbone).[1]

Clinical Notes: This muscle is commonly tight with patients suffering from bladder incontinence, prolapse of the uterus or bladder, and with prostatitis, rectal, and pelvic pain. This muscle often locks up and tightens after a fall onto the tailbone. It is often seen as significantly tight with a fractured coccyx, even many years later. When this muscle is tight, it restricts normal movement of the coccyx with the breath. The coccyx should extend and move outward like a "happy dog tail" on the inhale, and then move inward like a "bad dog tail" on the exhale. These mechanics are abnormal with tight coccygeus muscles and fascia.

The pelvic floor is important for many things, including stability at the lumbopelvic junction, stability among the organs of the reproductive system and abdomen, control of the lower body, continence of the bowel and bladder, healthy libido, and good neural control.

CREATE A STABLE FOUNDATION

Much like the foundation that holds up a house, the pelvic floor muscles provide the foundation for your body. The pelvis as a whole holds the core and upper body stable, like the base of a tree stabilizing its trunk. A solid foundation provides stability, and with stability you can build strength and power.

Overall, the strongest and fastest athletes are able to maintain good form throughout a race. They cross the finish line with perfect posture, not all bent over. Form and posture are largely created by a strong deep core, which creates a stable foundation. Occasionally a fast athlete will have a poor foundation, but often they will not be able to sustain their level of performance if their postural issues are not fixed. Just like a poor foundation under a house, they are placing significantly more load on their joints, and their body will not be able to endure. Sometimes athletes cannot withstand even one race, while other times they can go on for months or years with poor form before breaking down. However, poor foundation athletes, and poor foundation people in general, risk arthritis, degenerative disc disease, poor spinal alignment, incontinence, strains and sprains, and other medical diagnoses.

Again, *the pelvis is your foundation. Your entire upper and lower body rely on the stability of this foundation.* The upper body needs a stable place to rest on and the lower body needs a stable place to push off from and propel the body's movement. The pelvic floor muscles assist the pelvis to be stable.

What can happen if the pelvic floor muscles become weak? The pelvis will become unstable and the body will search for stability elsewhere, usually in a location above or below the pelvis. For example, I once worked with a patient diagnosed with "hamstring strain." Why was the hamstring strained? After releasing and restoring just some of her weak, tight, and dysfunctional pelvic floor muscles, the pain from her hamstring strain was gone. She felt better after just two visits. It is not uncommon for the hamstrings or adductors to become overworked with a tight and weak pelvic floor. By the way, if the pelvic floor is tight, *it is weak.*

If you can only lift your arm halfway, would you consider your arm strong? I would not, because the arm does not have full functional range. This lack of range can affect nearby joints, including the neck, elbow, and hand. Many, including myself, would argue that the lack of range at the shoulder affects joints even far from the shoulder, for example, the hip. Similarly, a weak and dysfunctional pelvic floor can affect joints both near and far.

The pelvic floor is not the only muscle group that stabilizes the pelvis. The transverse abdominis, which wraps around your belly like a girdle, and the gluteal musculature, the muscles that make up the buttocks, are also important. We will discuss the transverse abdominis muscle in the next chapter. The gluteus medius muscle is a huge stabilizer of the pelvis; however, I would not consider it as part of the deep core. The gluteus medius does assist in leveling the pelvis and prevents lateral shift of the pelvis, which can severely affect alignment. But unlike the deep core muscles, you can easily see the gluteus medius muscle. Furthermore, it is not a breathing muscle and is more easily turned on with simple exercises without conscious thought.

The pelvis is dynamic and susceptible to imbalances throughout the body. Anything above or below the pelvis can offset it, torquing and then compressing or shearing it one way or another. For example, a fallen arch of the foot will commonly cause the pelvis to drop and the hip to rotate internally on the side of the fallen arch. As a result, the pelvic floor becomes asymmetrical and is no longer as efficient as it was before the imbalance of the fallen arch.

When thinking about athletes such as runners or cyclists, an unstable pelvis would significantly reduce the power that could be generated from each arm or leg to propel them forward. One of a plethora of common problems I see and treat with cyclists is the inability to sit level on a bike; this problem is dynamic and involves the pelvic floor. Other common problems associated with weak and tight pelvic floor muscles include the following: numbness in the genitalia or down the leg; uncoordinated movements in one or both legs; lack of mobility in the hip, lower back, or pelvis; pain; and inability for the gluteal musculature to fire, or fire properly.

A balanced pelvis needs to be symmetrical. Think about a car: the axles need to be aligned along the drivetrain for optimum stability. If any components are misaligned, rotational, shear, tensile, or compression forces may interfere with the drivetrain or the axle, thus affecting the performance of the car. The result is a vehicle that will not drive as straight, fast, or smoothly as it should.

YOU CANNOT BYPASS THE PELVIS: IT IS PART OF YOUR ELECTRICAL CIRCUIT

You do not want the body to bypass the pelvic floor, as this will result in a delay in performance and recovery. The pelvic floor needs to be *turned on* and mobile for good neuronal (nerve) and blood flow. A delay in performance could mean a lack of agility, coordination, speed, timing, movement perfection, and ease of movement.

Think of the body as a branching electrical circuit. If one area is not firing, the body will find the next available path to complete the circuit. This is certainly not ideal, as your thigh musculature and lower back/sacrum are the next available paths, and will then be overworked and at risk for injury or weakened performance. Utilizing the less efficient path will also result in a lack of coordination and smoothness of motion. Bone is not the only tissue in the body that likes to be aligned! The ideal situation is for the tissues and joints to move smoothly together.

As another analogy, consider a snake. What if a quarter of the snake's body was locked up tight? The snake would not slither smoothly and sleekly, its appearance would be skewed, and its actions would not be as functional.

Or, think of an elderly person; perhaps they are unable to extend their back when going from sitting to standing, causing a delay before they can even stand straight. Or maybe they are slightly bent and immobile in some aspects of their spine when walking and appear stiff. These problems can affect youth also, but are statistically not as common.

Unfortunately, one can get "old" rather quickly. A car accident, for example, can create an abundance of problems in a split second, affecting multiple joints and tissues, leading to thousands of subsequent compensations. An eighteen-year-old involved in such a crash could feel sixty years old in one second as their body starts a plethora of new motor mechanics, bypassing many areas due to damage. Immediately, or years later, they will move very differently from their peers. What happens to us in life is what ages us, for good or bad.

I felt twenty-three when I had my first baby (I was actually thirty). After four months of no sleep, a poorly firing pelvic floor, and low back pain, I felt forty. Multiple musculoskeletal problems evolved and had to be reversed. I am happy to say that I now feel younger than my age once again.

Continence of urine and the bowel is another reason to keep the pelvic floor muscles *turned on* and coiling and recoiling. It has been known since the 1950s that the pelvic floor muscles help maintain continence, which is when Dr. Kegel developed the Kegel exercises. Kegel exercises are used to strengthen the pelvic floor to treat incontinence. Today, specialists prefer to simply call these exercises what they are — pelvic floor contractions. Numerous studies have proven the value of pelvic floor contractions in treating incontinence.

Even if you are continent (able to maintain a healthy flow of urine without accidents or wetting yourself), this is an important state to maintain. The pelvic floor is not the only muscle group responsible for continence, but it is one of primary importance. If your pelvic dynamics are weak for whatever reason, you will be more susceptible to episodes of incontinence.

STRESS INCONTINENCE

Stress incontinence is bladder leakage that happens with physical movement or activity. Coughing, sneezing, running, or jumping could initiate unwanted leakage. Sports with high pressure on the pelvic floor might make you more susceptible to stress incontinence. Running, jumping, volleyball, and crossfit put more stress on your pelvis and therefore increase your risk.[2]

Any musculoskeletal imbalance above or below the pelvis might also increase physical stress at the pelvic floor. A dropped foot arch, a shifting thoracic, scoliosis, rib misalignment, or even something as common as poor posture could cause incontinence. Hernias, pregnancy, and medical diagnoses affecting lung function are other common causes. All of these issues add to lumbopelvic instability and/or imbalance in the pelvic floor. Some research studies have referred to lumbopelvic instability as either wet or dry, "wet" meaning that a particular research group was leaking urine and "dry" meaning that they were not.[3]

Unfortunately, incontinence is not a rare condition. One study has shown that at least fifty percent of female collegiate athletes experience incontinence.[2] If you are planning on becoming a collegiate athlete or training like one, pay attention to this information and plan ahead for success. Furthermore, are you pregnant or planning to be? The mean prevalence of stress urinary incontinence during pregnancy is forty-one percent according to a research review.[4]

Half of female athletes and two out of five pregnant individuals is a large group of people who will benefit from *turning on* their pelvic floor. Some studies show higher or lower numbers, but either way, it is a lot of females. Training the pelvic floor has proven to be effective for treating incontinence and as a preventative measure against incontinence. Pelvic floor training should be used routinely, especially at the start of any pregnancy, to maintain continence. Furthermore, as you will learn, *all of the deep core muscles assist in maintaining continence.*

FUNCTION OF THE PELVIC FLOOR: CONTINENCE OF URINE

The pelvic floor assists in controlling continence of urine like a hand holding the nozzle of a hose. The specific muscles involved include the puborectalis muscle, which starts at the pubic bone and wraps around the backside of the rectum (see section Pubococcygeus), and the sphincter muscles of the urethra (compressor ureathra, urethral sphincter, and urethrovaginal sphincter).

FUNCTION OF THE PELVIC FLOOR: CONTINENCE OF BOWEL

The pelvic floor muscles, along with the anal sphincter muscles, also assist in holding back bowel movements and flatulence. The anal sphincter muscles are a ring of two muscles, the internal and external sphincter, at the opening of the anus. Depending on the amount of pressure needed to hold the bowel in, the sphincter muscles are *on* at all times to some degree. These muscles need to relax and lengthen in order to defecate. A Squatty Potty (a footstool that is placed around the toilet to raise the level of the knees while sitting) may assist with defecation. Raising the knees puts the hips and trunk at a shortened angle and elongates the angle at the sigmoid colon, allowing a bowel movement to exit more easily. Humans were designed to squat on nature's flora, which naturally allowed us to keep hip mobility and strength as well.

Like all deep core muscles, the pelvic floor muscles are breathing muscles. They are part of our body's internal pressure system. How are they assisting with the breath? As air comes in through the nose to fill the lungs, the pelvic floor lengthens. It works eccentrically, with a lengthening contraction. When I assess pelvic floors in the clinic, I ask the patient to take a deep breath in, and I feel for the pelvic floor to elongate and the tailbone to extend outward. I will feel this elongation even with restful inhalation in healthier pelvic floors.

Patients often ask how strong the pelvic floor needs to be. The strength that one needs depends on the amount of pressure coming into the lungs and abdominal cavity, gravity, weight of the body, and biomechanics and/or demands on the body. Imperfections and accommodations also affect the amount of strength needed, as do the dynamics of all of the deep core muscles. One example of an imperfection that would disrupt the dynamics of the deep core is restricted lower rib expansion. If your ribs are not expanding fully as you breathe, the pelvic floor will receive more of the pressure. More pressure could lead to incontinence. The expansion of your ribs allows for decreased compression forces at the pelvic floor and abdominal cavity with inhalation, for example, before a sneeze.

There are many causes of weak pelvic floors and incontinence. When the pelvic floor muscles are not *turned on* to their full capacity, the result can be a disruption in the pressure system. Sometimes simply being overly tight at the pelvic floor can cause muscles to misfire or fire poorly, which can cause incontinence of urine.

Surgery is another cause of incontinence and a weak pelvic floor. For example, after any cancer-related prostatectomy, physicians often tell their patients that they now have a risk for incontinence. They say the incontinence will clear up in a few weeks, within a few months, or in a few years. They go on to say there is always a risk that incontinence will not resolve. Some of my patients have told me they would rather have faced the cancer than deal with the incontinence they are now experiencing. I see patients with ongoing incontinence weeks, years, and often even decades after surgery. Ideally, I would see these patients *prior* to surgery for preventative care. Many states now offer pelvic floor therapy before and after prostatectomy surgery to teach pelvic floor contractions. Interestingly, I have seen more men being referred for prevention of incontinence following prostatectomy than women referred for prevention of incontinence during pregnancy. Either way, pelvic floor contractions are only one piece of the puzzle to prevent incontinence.

Why are some men incontinent after prostate surgery while others are not? Why are some women incontinent after or before giving birth while others are not? Surgery or pregnancy are often blamed for incontinence, sometimes rightly so. But sometimes it is not the surgery or pregnancy in and of itself that is responsible. My theory is that preexisting imbalances in the musculoskeletal system affect the pelvic floor directly or indirectly and play a role in the development of incontinence.

It is important to keep the body in good working order to withstand whatever life might throw at you. Some of my patients have had multiple musculoskeletal ailments prior to surgery that are simply ongoing or unresolved problems. Some examples include a weak core, poor breathing patterns, poor posture, atrophied gluteal musculature, poor range of motion at the hip and spine, scoliosis, scar tissue or adhesions, foot issues, hernias, diastasis rectus abdominis, bloating, and constipation. All of these imperfections can lead to increased chances of incontinence with or without surgery or pregnancy.

My focus with pelvic floor therapy involves alignment of the whole body. I prioritize not just the pelvic floor, but all deep muscles. When I see someone before prostate surgery or pregnancy, I will educate on the whole core and assist with strengthening weakness and perfecting posture and alignment. I will educate patients on their imperfections going into the surgery, how these are already affecting their mechanics and health, and how they can further affect the pelvis following surgery. Manual techniques and neuromuscular re-education will be specific and customized for each patient based on findings with evaluation.

PELVIC FLOOR STRENGTH AND MOBILITY:
SEXUAL HEALTH AND PLEASURE

Optimum pelvic health is necessary to maintain a healthy libido and to be able to achieve orgasm through intercourse or other sexual pleasures. In my clinical experience, patients report increased libido as a result of strengthening and improving mobility and alignment of the essential pelvic floor muscles. Like any deep core muscle, the pelvic floor muscles need to have full mobility to be able to fully lengthen and shorten, coil and recoil. Often, for multiple reasons, people develop myofascial trigger points and other fascial restrictions at their pelvic floor muscles, making intercourse painful.

A trigger point is a hyperirritable, sensitive, tender spot that is usually found within a taut band of skeletal muscle or fascia. Latent trigger points can cause functional restrictions without actively causing pain.[5] This is true in my experience, as I have seen a hundred times over. With palpation, a latent trigger point can cause local and referred pain. Furthermore, latent trigger points have been shown to have effects at the dorsal horn (one of the three grey columns of the spinal cord). Despite no pain being initially reported or felt, a latent trigger point can quickly become an active trigger point. An active trigger point has the same characteristics as a latent trigger point, but causes pain — referred or local or both — without palpation.

Referred pain is felt away from the site of the trigger point. Health care professionals and doctors will often mistake trigger point pain as being neurological in nature, meaning they assume the pain is coming from nerves at the central nervous system or the peripheral nervous system. However, trigger points themselves can and do cause neurological symptoms; they can entrap nerves and cause nerve pain (burning, numbness, tingling, itching, radiating). Trigger points can also change alignment of bony structures.

I use the term "neurological" loosely, as I believe you cannot always separate pathologies from musculoskeletal, neurological, orthopedic, joint, and vascular systems. I believe that all tissues work together. Many times you cannot have a problem with one and not the other. When someone says they only treat orthopedic disorders and not neurological disorders, this does not make any sense. You cannot have an arthritic knee (joint problem) without having nerve impairment (decreased proprioception, poor firing, uncoordinated movements) and muscle tissue impairments (muscle pain, poor muscle recruitment or motor unit activation, muscle dysfunction or weakness, tightness, imbalance).

Connective tissue restrictions often occur at the pelvic floor and can be felt between the skin and muscle. These restrictions may affect nerves, arteries, and veins, therefore indirectly affecting muscles, hips, and the pelvis. Connective tissue restrictions can cause pain; limited range of motion at the pelvic floor, pelvis, and hips; and decreased blood and nerve flow.

Pelvic floor restrictions frequently result in pain with intercourse, especially for females. I tend to see erectile dysfunction rather than pain in males. Dyspareunia is the medical term used to describe a sensation of pain while having intercourse. I have treated patients who have not been able to have pain-free sex for years and a few who have never had pain-free sex prior to therapy. Often the cause of pain for patients with dyspareunia is restrictions in the mobility of the pelvic floor. Moreover, due to tissue restrictions at the pelvic floor, the neurological response time of these patients is usually slower and less coordinated at the hips, pelvis, and lower back. This presentation is often what I refer to as a dysfunctional pelvis.

Most of the people I have treated are now able to happily state that they are pain-free as they engage in sex. This improvement is achieved by working with the patient in releasing, aligning, and strengthening the deep core. A variety of factors can disrupt the pelvic floor, either directly or indirectly. Direct influences might be trauma, birth, or surgery. Indirect influences might be foot drop or a weak hip. Sometimes restoring pain-free sex is as simple as releasing the pelvic floor muscles and then strengthening them. And for those who have no problems with their sex life, strengthening the deep core past the point of just functioning can make sex even better.

A more difficult cause of dyspareunia is sexual abuse. Often these people require seeing a psychologist who specializes in this area. With both a trained pelvic floor therapist and a psychologist, dyspareunia is most often successfully treated.

Another common clinical diagnosis is erectile dysfunction. Erectile dysfunction is not usually a physically painful condition in and of itself, but it does indicate that the pelvic area is affected. It can be very painful emotionally, and patients describe it as emasculating. Simply strengthening and releasing the pelvic floor muscles can often allow these patients to have an erection again. For some individuals to achieve an erection or to achieve an orgasm, the bulbospongiosus muscle and ischiocavernosus muscle (the external pelvic floor muscles) need to be released and *turned on* again.

Sometimes restoring pelvic floor mobility and strength is not done by addressing the pelvic floor directly. Often times limitations at the pelvic floor are from poor dynamics of other deep core muscles or musculoskeletal problems throughout the body.

PELVIC FLOOR MOBILITY AND STRENGTH PREVENT PROLAPSE

Pelvic organ prolapse is the downward descent of the pelvic organs (uterus, bladder, rectum, intestines, sigmoid colon) from their resting position. Fascial and muscular restrictions often contribute to the issue, specifically at the coccygeus muscles (the back muscles of the pelvic floor). If prolapse is a problem, the pelvic floor muscles will have to be released. A specialist will be able to assist with the proper exercises and manual bodywork to accomplish this. Studies show significant improvements in prolapse with pelvic floor therapy; grades of prolapse can change.[6,7] Therapy can also prevent the need for surgery.

Strengthening and restoring the other deep core muscles will help with prolapse problems. The abdominal muscles, specifically the transverse abdominis, will also need to be strengthened, as the abdominal muscles help to lift the uterus and bladder. Posture and alignment will also need to be restored.

HOW DO YOU *TURN ON* THE PELVIC FLOOR MUSCLES?

Turning on the pelvic floor muscles requires three steps: identification, activation, and strengthening. The first step is to know how to identify these muscles. Below is a list of tests to assist with this. After the tests, I have written some pearls of wisdom on what to look for when activating the pelvic floor muscles. A little knowledge on normal and abnormal is helpful. One can use simple range of motion exercises, listed as cues, to strengthen different regions of the pelvic floor or the pelvic floor as a whole. The cues/exercises allow one to focus on a specific fiber group, or on the pelvic floor muscles as a whole.

Keep in mind that, because the pelvis is dynamic, any body structure above or below the pelvis can make the pelvic floor weak, imbalanced, or unstable. Note that many manual treatment techniques activate the pelvic muscles and restore range of motion and strength without actually *turning the deep core on*. Meaning, a thorough exam evaluating alignment and correcting imbalances with special techniques can sometimes improve or assist in activation of the pelvic floor muscles without any deep core exercises, as the deep core often fires/activates when it is positioned for success (with correct biomechanics and alignment).

It is nice to know if the deep core muscles are on or off and if they have normal range of motion. If you don't know there is problem, why and how would you fix it? And how do you know if it is fixed?

HOW CAN YOU IDENTIFY IF THE PELVIC FLOOR MUSCLES ARE TURNED ON?

Finger Test

Inside your vagina (on all sides of it) or inside your rectum (on all sides of it), you can feel the pelvic floor, with the bulk of the muscle being on the back side near your tailbone (coccyx) and less bulk at the pubic bone. If you are inserting a finger into the rectum, you will feel a pair of circular rings of muscle called the sphincter muscles before you reach the pelvic floor. Assessing the pelvic floor rectally can be tricky and uncomfortable if you have limited shoulder or spine mobility. I would recommend wearing a glove and putting lubricant on the glove before assessing rectally!

Prior to a vaginal assessment, make sure your hands are washed. Start by lying on your side and try to bring the knees up in a bent position towards your chest. Try and relax all other muscles. Make sure your big gluteus muscles are not contracting, relax your abdominal muscles, and relax your inner thigh muscles. Insert a finger into the vagina at least up to the first knuckle. The first muscle you will feel on all sides of your finger is the puborectalis muscle. If you go further laterally towards your hips to your right and left side, you will feel the iliococcygeus muscle. If you reach back towards your rectum, you will feel your tailbone and coccygeus muscle on either side of the tailbone. The coccygeus muscle can be hard to assess for some with less back/pelvis mobility and short fingers.

Attempt to contract the pelvic floor while inside the rectum or vagina. Use some cues while contracting. Try using the instruction, "bring your tailbone to your pubic bone and then up towards your head." Note the mobility of the pelvic floor. Is it moving? Note the tension of the pelvic floor. Is it contracting or changing tension?

Once you have identified the pelvic floor muscles, you can use cues to target certain muscle groups. For the anterior fibers (the puborectalis), you can say, "bring your clitoris to your pubic bone," and place your fingers in the vagina toward the pubic bone. For the middle fibers (the iliococcygeus), you can imagine, "bring a marble up your vagina towards your head." For the posterior fibers, you can use the cue, "tuck your tailbone/coccyx under your tummy like a dog tucks his tail under his tummy when he has done something bad." We will discuss more cues in a later section of this chapter.

Partner Test

Another way to identify and test the strength of the pelvic floor muscles is through intercourse. Try to identify these muscles by squeezing your partner's penis, or a dildo, with your internal pelvic floor muscles. During any position in intercourse, tighten your pelvic floor muscles and ask if your partner can feel it. Also — ask yourself.

GRADE YOURSELF with finger and/or partner test:

0 — Unable to feel a squeeze or contraction.

1 — Able to feel a contraction.

2 — Able to feel a contraction with some strength behind it.

3 — Able to feel a contraction and resist a penis/dildo from being pulled out of the vagina.

Urine Test

One way you may try to test the strength of the pelvic floor is to begin to urinate and then try to stop the flow of urine midstream. If your body is functioning correctly, this should be easy to do. It is *not* recommended that you do this exercise everyday, because you want to relax those muscles to allow normal urination. You do NOT want to train a bad habit. Doing this once a week, however, will not be enough to change your neuromuscular patterning. Neuromuscular changes require mass practice, as discussed later in this chapter.

GRADE YOURSELF:

0 — You cannot stop the flow of urine.

1 — You can try to stop the flow of urine midstream with some leaks.

2 — You can stop the flow of urine midstream without leaking.

Tailbone Test

Lie on your back with your knees bent and touching each other. Place your feet flat on the ground. Place your finger on your tailbone, the end of your spine, the bony prominence just before your rectum. Try to activate your pelvic floor muscles — you should feel movement of your tailbone. You can also place your fingers on either side of your tailbone, and again you should feel tension under your fingers with contraction of the pelvic floor. The movement should be upward (towards the head) and forward (towards the pubic bone). If the tailbone is moving, this is a sign that the pelvic floor muscles are contracting and have mobility.

Balloon Test

Can you blow up a balloon? Start with a larger balloon and then move on to smaller balloons. Larger balloons require less pelvic floor strength. You should be able to easily blow up any size balloon. If you are unable to, this is a sign that your pelvic floor is weak or potentially not turned on.

ISOLATING THE MOVEMENT TO THE PELVIC FLOOR MUSCLES: ACTIVATION

With each exercise, try to *isolate the contraction* to just your pelvic floor area while quieting all the other muscles of your pelvis (commonly the muscles of the buttocks, the long muscles of the legs, and the abdominal muscles will want to assist). Start by *lying down*. This takes gravity out of the picture, as well as any imbalances in your body that may be amplified in other positions. Place a pillow under your knees and head as needed to *support your structure*. *Take your breath out of the picture,* as breath can cause more muscle confusion. Start by taking a deep breath in and a partial breath out. Now *hold your breath* and contract your pelvic floor muscles. This way you can *feel more* and your body doesn't need to coordinate as much movement.

Visualize your tailbone moving to the back side of your pubic bone, like a dog tucking his tail underneath his body towards his belly. "Go tailbone… past your rectum… past your vagina/testicles… past your clitoris/penis… to the back side of your pubic bone and up towards your head." Then, reverse the action and think of lengthening your pelvic floor. Just like a bicep curl, don't just drop out, but rather control the descent. Imagine a happy dog, with its tail coming up. This is the same direction you want to move your tailbone as you lengthen your pelvic floor. "From the back of the pubic bone… past your clitoris/penis… past your vagina/testicles… past your rectum… to your tailbone." You might also want to *close your eyes* to feel and "see" more. You will be amazed how much more you can feel with your eyes closed.

People often try too hard to activate these muscles on demand. But it is best to try to think "local and light" when you begin. You don't want everything firing immediately. We are trying to isolate the muscle, especially if it is weak. The desired muscle will never have its turn if it is weak and everything fires. Your muscle might be like a weak soccer player who is confronted by "ball hogs" who are not giving the newbie a turn, and who never gets to develop the skills or strength to play. Let your muscle play and get stronger so the team will be stronger.

DON'T RECRUIT ALL OF YOUR ABDOMINAL MUSCLES WHEN ACTIVATING THE PELVIC FLOOR MUSCLES

You should not see your abdominal muscles (obliques or rectus abdominis) fire when isolating the pelvic floor muscles. What if you contracted your obliques and rectus abdominis every time while doing a pelvic floor contraction? This would compress your abdominal content, causing unwanted pressure on your pelvic floor. Certainly this is not an ideal outcome when you are trying to decompress the pelvic floor. If you give your child a juice box in the car and they squeeze the box too hard, the pressure will cause leakage out of the straw. Squeezing all of the abdominal muscles could eventually lead to the leaking of urine through the urethra. It could also cause pressure toward the stomach and esophagus leading to GERD. This is a good reason not to walk around with all your abdominal muscles contracted to "look good." You would not want all of the abdominal muscles constantly contracting and compressing so that your abdominal contents spill onto your pelvic floor or your stomach content is pushed up through the esophagus.

PELVIC FLOOR MUSCLES FIRE WITH YOUR TRANSVERSE ABDOMINIS

Your pelvic floor needs to contract in isolation from your big abdominal muscles, BUT in conjunction with your transverse abdominis. You will learn more about the transverse abdominis in the next chapter. Again, I repeat, it is normal for the transverse abdominis to activate with the pelvic floor. When isolating the pelvic floor, you might feel a co-contraction of the traverse abdominis. It is often subtle. However, one should not see the obliques and rectus abdominis firing while training the pelvic floor in isolation.

HOW DO YOU KNOW IF YOUR PELVIC FLOOR MUSCLES ARE *TURNED ON* AND FUNCTIONING PROPERLY?

The pelvic floor should have movement. You should be able to *feel the movement*. You should feel both a *forward and upward* movement on the shortening of the muscle and a *downward and backward* movement on lengthening of the muscle. If either one of these movements is missing, it is a sign of a weak or dysfunctional (not moving with normal mechanics) pelvic floor. Just like moving your arm or leg, you should be able to move at *multiple speeds*, slow to fast. And the movement should be controlled, not jerky, but rather *smooth and fluid* and with ease.

Another characteristic of a *turned on* pelvic floor is its ability to *resist pressure.* You should feel pressure of the pelvic floor muscles around your finger and/or around a dildo and/or penis. In other words, the pelvic floor should have some strength behind it. It should also be able to *resist gravity;* you should be able to *feel this muscle contracting in all positions* (sitting, standing, walking, squatting). These are tasks in which the pelvic floor has to work harder than when you are lying down.

A healthy, *turned on* pelvic floor has symmetry. You should feel that the pelvic floor is symmetrical left and right and front and back. Your pelvic floor should have an equal range of motion, ease, and speed of movement on all sides.

HOW DO YOU KNOW IF THE PELVIC FLOOR MUSCLES ARE STRONG?

Strong pelvic floor muscles will have all the qualities and characteristics of being *turned on,* as listed above. Generally speaking, you should be able to easily hold a pelvic floor contraction for at least thirty seconds with some resistance. Resistance might include gravity (standing), weight of the body plus impact (running, jumping, squatting), pressure (holding your breath or a combination of movements). Your pelvic floor has to be able to withstand the daily forces you request of it. You have to *strengthen it for your needs and wants.* In terms of speed, you should be able to easily do ten full contractions in ten seconds. A full contraction means going through the full range of motion of the pelvic floor. Just like a full squat, go for full shortening and lengthening of the muscle fiber — *do not cut it short on either end.*

WHAT ARE THE SIGNS YOU ARE *TURNED OFF?*

The same method that determines if you are *turned on* will also tell you if you are turned off. You will know that you are turned off if you are unable to stop your flow of urine, if you are unable to feel a contraction with your partner test, or if you cannot feel your pelvic floor muscles contract with the finger test. If you are not turned on, you will not be able to move the pelvic floor forward and up or backward and down. You will not feel movement at the pelvic floor, or you will not feel full movement. Pelvic floor movement will not have the ability to go different speeds. Movement of the pelvic floor might be jerky and uncoordinated, delayed, and/or sluggish. You might not feel any pressure, or minimal pressure, around your finger or around a dildo or penis. The pelvic floor might not be able to contract against gravity — you might have the inability to perform a pelvic floor contraction while sitting, standing, walking, or squatting. You might also feel asymmetry of the pelvic floor. Another sign that your pelvic floor muscles are not functioning properly is that you are unable to have an orgasm.

ANOTHER POSSIBILITY:

YOU ARE STUCK IN A *TURNED ON* POSITION

You might not be able to feel any movement or contraction because the pelvic floor muscles are stuck in a shortened or lengthened position. When the muscle is locked "on" it is not coiling and recoiling, shortening and lengthening. If the pelvic floor is immobile, it is weak. In this case, the muscle is *turned on, but not working with full, functional mobility.* One way to address this is to ask yourself if there is any movement at all. Compare the front, back, left, and right sides of your pelvic floor. You should be able to feel movement in all areas, and not just a contraction or tightening.

To know if you have full mobility, you will have to ask a trained pelvic floor therapist. *It is hard to determine normal mobility without the pure experience of working with many pelvic floors.* Nevertheless, you should be able to assess if there is mobility. A normal pelvic floor contraction should result in a cranio-ventral shift of the pelvic organs. In other words, you should feel the movement go from the tailbone to the pubic bone and up towards your head. You can feel this kinesthetically (through the senses), by feel with just your fingers, or through thought directed at your pelvis. Similarly, the lower back portion of the bladder will be lifted towards the head and the front of your body with a pelvic floor contraction. This can be seen on ultrasound imaging.

Some abnormal responses can be seen with ultrasound-guided imaging in a clinic. One example of an abnormal response is excessive movement of the bladder during spinal loading (coughing, jumping, or running). The bladder might move down or to either side rather than up and to the front of the pelvis. With imaging, no lift of the caudo-dorsal (bottom back) portion of the bladder can be seen upon an attempted contraction.

Imaging is not always needed, but it can be very helpful to connect the body to the brain. My patients have really appreciated this technology, as now they can see their deep core. It is amazing, ultrasound-guided therapy for activation of your deep core!

Another type of abnormal response is an over-activation of synergistic muscles (abdominal bracing and/or posterior tilt). This occurs when other muscles are recruited instead of the pelvic floor muscles or in conjunction with the pelvic floor muscles. Other muscles commonly used when asked to activate the pelvic floor are the internal and external obliques and rectus abdominis, along with the adductors or rotators of the hip. Sometimes it is normal for all of these muscles to be recruited, but for the purpose of strengthening the pelvic floor, you should be able to isolate just the pelvic floor muscles. We must make sure that the pelvic floor muscles are turned on and working with full capacity (range of motion and strength). As mentioned previously, the one exception is the transverse abdominis; when the pelvic floor muscles contract, the transverse abdominis should contract too. If this co-contraction does not exist, something is wrong.

Another abnormality is the inability to fully relax after a contraction. This may lead to shortened pelvic floor muscles, or could be a sign that the muscles are already shortened. Shortened pelvic floor muscles could indicate a lack of blood flow and a lack of axonal (nerve) flow. If the pelvic floor is not able to relax or lengthen, it will not be as adaptable or responsive, it will fatigue easily, and it will become weak and tight. The inability to relax can also lead to trigger points and pain with intercourse, as well as pelvic pain, abdominal pain, or groin pain. This sort of pain is not only dysfunctional, it can also affect the mechanics above and below the pelvis resulting in abnormal breathing, difficulty defecating, dyspareunia, and other issues.

HOW DO YOU KNOW IF THE PELVIC FLOOR IS TOO TIGHT?

Sometimes, even when the pelvic floor muscles are firing, you might not feel movement. This is likely the result of muscle and fascia tightness. Identifying the cause of the tightness is important in order to gain back full range of motion. If tightness exists, I would recommend seeing an experienced pelvic floor therapist to learn how to release these muscles. Before working on strength, you might need to work on regaining a normal range of motion and alignment.

Tightness can also spread to other joints. For example, if your shoulder is tight, you might suddenly find that it is hard to move your neck, elbow, or wrist. Similarly, if your pelvic floor is tight, it can restrict sacroiliac joint mobility (which links the lower spine and pelvis) and movement of the hip.

Not only will you want the tightness released at the pelvic floor, you will need to fix the cause of why the muscles are tight. The cause of the tightness is not always so direct, as it could be as distant as the cranium. Sometimes the cause is primarily psychological in nature; certain muscles will respond to emotional or psychological stresses and do not always release until the psyche and/or emotion has been treated. This is where you want the expertise of an experienced pelvic floor therapist who uses a whole body approach to treat their patients.

GETTING *TURNED ON* AND
STRENGTHENING THE PELVIC FLOOR

Here are some techniques to both *turn on* the pelvic floor muscles and to strengthen them if they are already *on*. These exercises are in the form of cues. *Cues* are verbal prompts that may be said aloud or silently within your mind. Some may work for you and others might not have significance for your brain-to-body connection. Try the following verbal cues to both activate and strengthen your pelvic floor.

PELVIC FLOOR ACTIVATION EXERCISES WITH VERBAL CUING

These exercises are meant to isolate and fire different muscle fiber groups (front, middle and back) of your pelvic floor. When activating the pelvic floor, you should feel movement near and around the genitalia, pubic bone, tailbone, and rectum. Your pelvic floor muscles connect to the tailbone and the rectum. Before working on strengthening these muscles, you should be able to identify them using the aforementioned tests and knowledge and these cueing exercises.

Cues to Activate and Strengthen the Front Fibers

- Nod the clitoris.
- Move the coccyx (tailbone) to the pubic bone and nod the clitoris.
- Lift the base of the penis.
- Move the clitoris towards the pubic bone, up further, as far as you can bring it.

Cues to Activate the Middle Fibers (Mainly the Iliococcygeus)

- Bring a marble up the vagina.
- Bring the labia together and up (also working bulbospongiosus).
- Bring the sit bones to the pubic bone (working ischiocavernosus and transverse superficialis).
- Bring the tail bone to the pubic bone.
- Lift the testicles up.

Cues to Activate the Back Fibers (Mainly the Coccygeus)

- Move the tailbone to the head.
- Hold in stool with the sphincter muscles.
- Stop gas from coming out.
- Bring the tailbone to the pubic bone or clitoris.
- Like a bad dog, move the tailbone toward the pubic bone and up towards the head.

Cues to Activate All Muscle Groups Together

- Bring the tailbone to the pubic bone, nod the clitoris, and lift up towards the head from the clitoris.
- Bring the tailbone to the pubic bone, lift the base of the penis and move it up further.
- Go up the elevator (one floor at a time): contract the pelvic floor muscles while directing them forward and up. Then go down the elevator (one floor at a time): slowly lengthen the pelvic floor from pubic bone to coccyx.

Noises and Faces to Turn On or Shorten the Pelvic Floor Muscles

- Make an "mmm" sound.
- Laugh.
- Smile.

Noises and Faces to Turn Off or Lengthen the Pelvic Floor Muscles

- Make an "sss" sound.
- Put a "frown" on your face.

You can also use the transverse abdominis activating exercises in the next chapter to help turn on your pelvic floor muscles or identify them. With normal biomechanics, when the pelvic floor contracts, so does the transverse abdominis and vice versa.

First make sure you are *turned on* with above tests, knowledge, and cuing. Then get your baseline! Determine your endurance; how long can you hold a pelvic floor contraction before it fatigues or weakens greater than fifty percent? I like to start with this number and do ten repetitions of pelvic floor contractions six times a day.

How do you know when you have fatigued fifty percent or more? Assess the amount of fatigue by feeling the contraction with your fingers or kinesthetically (body awareness of movement and tension). When you let go of the contraction, was there anything to let go of? If you felt no change or movement, you fatigued one hundred percent. You might notice that you lost a percentage of the strength you were originally able to hold/feel when you contracted your pelvic floor. It is like lifting a weight with a bicep curl. When you start to fatigue, it is harder to lift to the end range. The pelvic floor form is lost when the lift lightens, the amount of contractile strength is lessened, or the mobility lessens.

Which cue or activation exercise should you use? You might find you can contract the pelvic floor better (stronger, longer, more fluidly, or with more mobility) with some cues. Also, you might notice that some of the muscle fibers of the pelvic floor, front versus back for example, might be weaker than the others. Or maybe the right is stronger than the left. I would choose one cue from each muscle fiber group and one cue to activate all the muscle fibers together. Therefore, you will have four exercises to do for six sets of ten repetitions a day. Ideally you will not do these all at one time, nor should you be able to; that is two hundred and forty pelvic floor contractions, ideally done throughout the day.

What position should one start in? For example, say you can hold a contraction of the pelvic floor for five seconds while lying down and then it fatigues greater than fifty percent. Then you would do five-second holds for ten repetitions while lying down, six times a day. If you attempt these exercises while sitting and cannot feel a contraction or activate against gravity, continue to work in anti-gravity positions until your strength and endurance improve. A thirty-second hold in any position is a good indicator that you are ready to try something more challenging. For example, you might move from lying flat to sitting, then sitting to standing, and standing to squatting. Making the position harder might involve adding gravity, weight, more dynamic movements, and/or momentum. Work your way through this positional progression of pelvic floor strengthening:

• Take your breath out of the biomechanical equation to assist in identifying and initiating the coordination of the deep core. When you hold your breath, movement becomes quieted and you can better feel the pelvic floor. Obviously you need to breathe, so incorporate the breath back into the exercises when you can easily identify the pelvic floor.
• Get into horizontal positions, such as lying on the back, stomach, or side, so part of your body is supported by the ground. Remember that the pelvic floor muscles and all of the deep core muscles work to stabilize you. Take that job away while re-activating or iso-

lating the pelvic floor. Horizontal positions take the weight of the upper body off of the pelvis.

- When you are able to do deep core exercises in horizontal positions, it is time to progress to vertical positions. Vertical positions stack your body weight and tend to make activation of the pelvic floor more difficult. Furthermore, vertical positions do not offer as much support as lying on the ground and tend to add to poor mechanics that might already exist in the body.

- Sitting is normally harder than lying down because you have added both gravity and your weight on top of your pelvis. You add and potentially exponentially compound more musculoskeletal issues.

- Standing is harder than sitting because now you have no surface to sit on — the surface can act with the pelvic floor to support the pelvis. Imbalances from the lower extremities can now change the dynamics of the pelvic floor.

- Weight is harder than no weight.

- Dynamic positions are harder than stable positions.

- Walking is harder than standing because it requires multiple movements within the body and environment.

- Running is more dynamic than walking — forces are greater and, in essence, imbalances within the body and environment can also be greater.

Remember, misalignment and posture also impact the ability of the pelvic floor to fire. The deep core fires best when the spine is aligned. Musculoskeletal imbalances at the torso and extremities can change the spinal myofascial and bony alignment. A well-functioning pelvic floor will assist in musculoskeletal alignment. Also keep in mind that this is a *general* list of progression. There are cases where, for example, individuals can fire the deep core in the most progressive position listed, but not while lying down.

A PLEASURABLE WAY TO STRENGTHEN THE PELVIC FLOOR:
SEX

Sex is a great way to have fun while turning on the pelvic floor and transverse abdominis muscles. Masturbation and the use of sex toys such as dildos or vibrators are also ways to turn on your pelvic floor muscles. Sexual activity and sex toys offer a way to feel the muscles, to manipulate them, and to make them want to activate and participate. I recommend vibrating dildos with clitoral stimulus versus just one or the other. Vibration is a form of extra stimulus and a tool that therapists use to manipulate and activate muscles in general.

Sex is also important to maintain the ability to have sex. Vaginas can develop stenosis, a condition in which the vagina grows together and the vaginal canal closes, narrows, or shortens. Stenosis can omit the ability for penile, dildo, or digital penetration. I have seen this happen in my patients. The body does morph, and this is just one way it can do this. Stenosis can also be a complication of radiation "therapy." However, I have seen stenosis of the vagina from simple lack of use.

I strongly recommend sex and masturbation, as compliance and consistency is better when learning how to activate the pelvic floor muscles. Both sex and masturbation assist in getting turned on and turning others on.

Make sex a workout to add emphasis to the muscles. Just because you are having sex doesn't mean your muscles are *turned on* or working to their full capacity. I have felt many extremely weak pelvic floor muscles in very sexually active people. Focusing on the movement of the pelvic floor while participating in sexual activity is important. Mindful movement! You can actually do sets of contractions while masturbating or having intercourse.

It all depends where you are with the strength of your pelvic floor muscles as far as what sexual activity is going to do for you. What's sex doing for your pelvic floor? Activating it, strengthening it, coordinating it, bulking it up, giving you mobility, improving your libido — go find out! Or nothing!?

INCORPORATE PELVIC FLOOR MUSCLE
EXERCISES INTO YOUR LIFESTYLE

If you run, you can coordinate the pelvic floor with your breathing, lengthening the pelvic floor muscles with the inhale and contracting the pelvic floor muscles with the exhale. Another option would be to just contract the pelvic floor for "x" amount of time while running.

If you do yoga, you can coordinate the pelvic floor with every breath, forcing elongation with the inhale and shortening with the exhale. Or contract the pelvic floor muscles while holding certain positions.

If you lift weights, you can add the pelvic floor to your upper extremity, lower extremity, or core strengthening exercises. Just consciously contract the pelvic floor with each exercise.

Make the pelvic floor a part of your life. Too often we sit, and when we sit the pelvic floor can turn off as its job is taken over by the surface we sit on. The muscle becomes less responsive. So actively *turn yourself on* daily.

ANOTHER WAY TO STRENGTHEN THE PELVIC FLOOR: BREATH

Your pelvic floor muscles are breathing muscles and breathing is another way to strengthen them. The pelvic floor is a breathing muscle in its ability to assist you with inhalation, exhalation, vocalization, and restoring the pressure system. Singing is being acknowledged as another recreational way to strengthen the pelvic floor muscles.[8]

What is a normal breath? And what is the normal job of the pelvic floor while breathing? When you take a restful breath in, the pelvic floor eccentrically contracts/lengthens and descends downward (relative to the head when standing). Just like lowering the arm during a bicep curl, this is a lengthening movement. When you exhale, air is pushed up and out, and the pelvic floor shortens/concentrically contracts. The role of the pelvic floor and breathing with dynamic movements is less studied, and a topic of debate among physical therapists. When running, I believe the same movement happens, but with a stronger effort at the pelvic floor with both inhale and exhale. In addition, I feel the pelvic floor works in a more shortened and *on* position while running. I believe it cannot come to end range length or shortening as it has to work to both stabilize and breathe. The pelvic floor has to be dynamic and is constantly adjusting for the pressure that is placed on it.

MASS PRACTICE MAKES PERFECT

As you learn to make changes in your deep muscles and motor patterning, you will need to begin mass practice. Mass practice consists of doing something as specific as six sets of ten pelvic floor movements per day while re-enacting all of the normal motions that we go through in life. This will be slightly different for each person, but most of us will be practicing familiar patterns like squatting, walking, or sitting in a healthful manner. If your pelvic floor muscles are too weak, you will have to progress to such tasks.

SIX SETS OF TEN REPETITIONS

Remember, retraining the deep core muscles takes mass practice, six sets of ten repetitions in every position or function you want them to succeed in assisting you. You have to train the deep muscles to be sport-specific or specific to the activities of your daily living. For example, you cannot just exercise the pelvic floor muscles while sitting if you want them to work with your normal activities of daily living (walking, standing, squatting, running, body building, etc.). Squatting, running, and jumping will require a stronger pelvic floor; you need to train the pelvic floor for the load it will need to handle.

In general, things that help to take stress off of the pelvic floor include good alignment; symmetry; having the extremities free from the core and vice versa, as discussed previously; and having the other deep core muscles functioning and acting within their full ability of range, strength, and neuromuscular control. Inversion and rest, although commonly missed, are also important to your muscles and overall health.

You should maintain strength and mobility in a few other muscles of the pelvis that are rarely discussed. These muscles are the ischiocavernosus, transverse superficialis, and bulbospongiosus. See figures at the beginning of this chapter for anatomical location. The functions of these muscles are discussed below, along with cues for how they can be *turned on*.

Ischiocavernosus

Location/Insertion: Above sit bone on inner side (ramus of ischium) to clitoris in females and to crux of penis in males.

Function/Action: In females, clenches/closes the vagina; in males, empties the urethra and compresses the penis (to assist with erections).

Bulbospongiosus

Location: In females, borders the clitoris and vagina. In males, surrounds the base of the penis.[1]

Function/Action: In females, assists in clenching the vagina and in having an orgasm. In males, assists with emptying the bladder and having an erection.

Clinical Notes: If males are having difficulty with erections or emptying urine, I have them massage from the shaft of the penis to the tip of the penis after urination. This assists with releasing the fascia and the bulbospongiosus muscle while also increasing circulation to the shaft of the penis.

Cues to Turn On the Ischiocavernosus and Bulbospongiosus

• Bring the sit bones to the pubic bone.
• Bring the labia together.
• Move leg out, use cue "bring the labia together," then bring leg in.
• Lift the base of the penis.

Transverse Superficialis

Origin: Ischial tuberosity (sit bones).

Location/Insertion: Perineal body (central tendinous point) between rectum and vagina in females and rectum and scrotum in males.

Function/Action: Supports the pelvic floor and the expulsion of the last drop of urine in both sexes. Supports the expulsion of semen in males.

Cue to Turn On the Transverse Superficialis

- Cue "bring sit bones together." You should feel tension between the sit bones on either side of the perineal body.
- To isolate, squat at a ninety-nine degree angle with your back against a wall (chair position). Cue "bring sit bones together." The gluteus maximus will stretch, making the transverse superficialis more readily felt.

OTHER TYPES OF STRENGTHENING

The exercises in this chapter, just like any strengthening exercise, can be modified to fit your needs. Maybe you want to focus on coordination of the pelvic floor muscles while doing "elevator" pelvic floor contractions. Focus on slowly contracting the pelvic floor one level at a time, really focusing on getting to the top floors. The "top floors" can be thought of as the front fibers and as stronger contractions (getting more muscle fibers recruited with each floor). Then, slowly lower from the top floor to the bottom floor, which would be the pelvic floor in its most lengthened position.

Another example might be power or resistance training. You can use a dildo and try to pull it out while holding a pelvic floor contraction. This becomes a game of tug-of-war, thus providing resistance training. Or you can use vaginal weights, holding them in the vagina while doing activities of daily living (walking, squatting, laundry). Or you can buy dildos that measure strength to some degree and challenge yourself that way. You can also progress to harder positions, as noted previously in this chapter.

THIS IS SO DIFFERENT

You will notice that the exercises described above do not look like the typical diagrams of strengthening exercises in the gym, and they are not. All of these pelvic floor muscles fire non-stop; they are being used for breathing and posture, and are trained a little differently for that reason. Although you cannot quite see these muscles and they are not obvious to you yet, I hope you are "seeing" them more clearly as you read and experiment with them. However, if you still cannot get the pelvic floor muscles firing, or you do not know for certain if you are doing the pelvic floor contractions correctly, I would strongly recommend seeing a pelvic floor therapist. You may be under the impression that your body is operating perfectly with the exception of your pelvic floor issues, but it is highly unlikely. When the pelvic floor muscles are dysfunctional, there is often a plethora of musculoskeletal issues going on.

REFERENCES
1. Netter FH. *Atlas of Human Anatomy.* 7th ed. Elsevier; 2018.
2. Dockter M, Kolstad AM, Martin KA, Schiwal LJ. Prevalence of urinary incontinence: A comparative study of collegiate female athletes and non-athletic controls. *Journal of Women's Health Physical Therapy.* 2007;31:12-17.

doi:10.1097/01274882-200731010-00003

3. Lee D, Lee L. Stress urinary incontinence — a consequence of failed load transfer through the pelvis? Presented at: 5th World Interdisciplinary Congress on Low Back and Pelvic Pain; November 2004; Melbourne, Australia.

4. Sangsawang B, Sangsawang N. Stress urinary incontinence in pregnant women: A review of prevalence, pathophysiology, and treatment. International Urogynecology Journal. 2013;24:901-912. doi:10.1007/s00192-013-2061-7

5. Travell JG, Simons DG. *Myofascial Pain and Dysfunction: The Trigger Point Manual.* Williams and Wilkins; 1983.

6. Hagen S, Stark D, Glazener C, Sinclair L, Ramsay I. A randomized controlled trial of pelvic floor muscle training for stages I and II pelvic organ prolapse. *International Urogynecology Journal and Pelvic Floor Dysfunction.* 2009;20:45-51. doi:10.1007/s00192-008-0726-4

7. Stüpp L, Resende APM, Oliveira E, et al. Pelvic floor muscle training for treatment of pelvic organ prolapse: An assessor-blinded randomized controlled trial. *International Urogynecology Journal.* 2011;22:1233-1239. doi:10.1007/s00192-011-1428-x

8. Bedekar N. Pelvic floor muscle activation during singing: A pilot study. *Journal of the Association of Chartered Physiotherapists in Women's Health.* 2012;110:27-32.

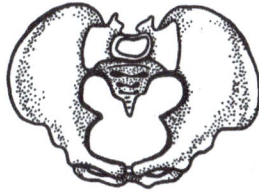

TRANSVERSE ABDOMINIS

Just look at the transverse abdominis! It's massive! It is your dynamic human girdle. The transverse abdominis spans your entire lower body from back to front, on all sides. In Figure 3.1, the rectus abdominis, internal oblique, and external oblique muscles have been removed to expose the transverse abdominis muscle (in pink/red) and its aponeurosis (a fibrous membrane that serves as a form of fascia; in white).

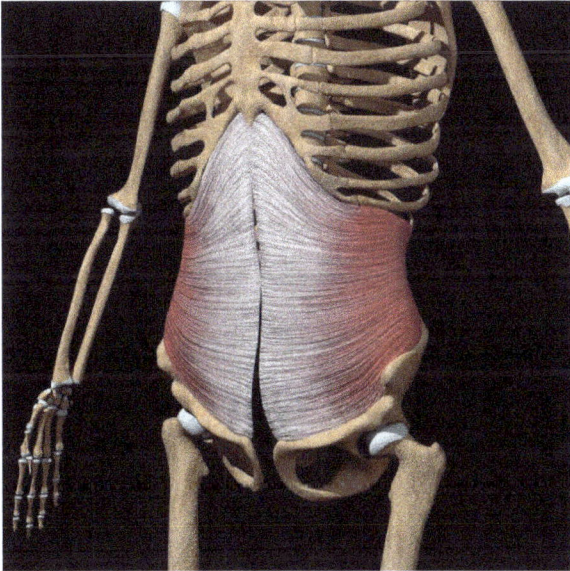

Figure 3.1. The transverse abdominis.
From MadiGraphic/*Shutterstock.com.*

Your rectus abdominis (or "six-pack") is the abdominal muscle at the front and center of your abdomen (see Figure 3.2). The muscles along the sides of your "six-pack" are the external obliques, internal obliques, and transverse abdominis. There is also another muscle just above the pubic bone called the pyramidalis. There are five abdominal muscles, but we are mainly interested in the deepest of these muscles — the transverse abdominis.

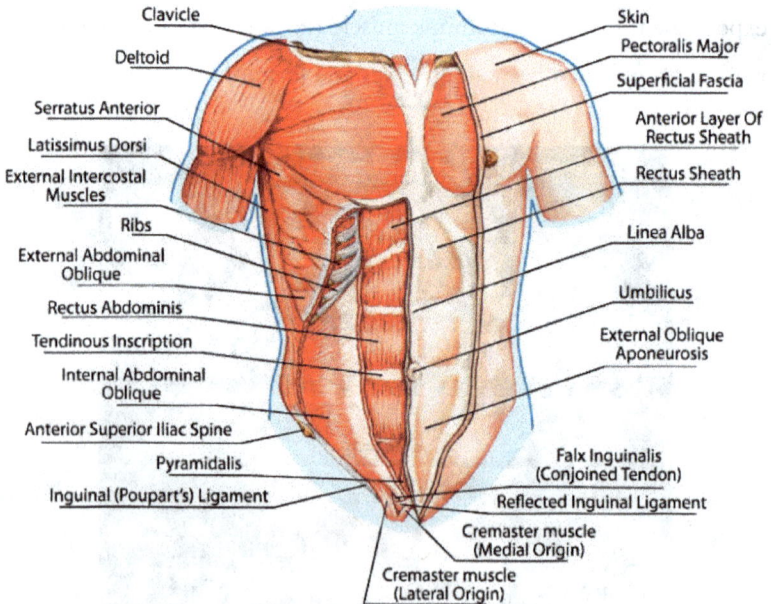

Figure 3.2. Abdominal anatomy.
From Stihii/*Shutterstock.com*.

RECTUS ABDOMINIS

The rectus abdominis is not literally a six-pack. It is an eight-pack; there are eight muscle belly groups that make up the rectus abdominis muscles. The rectus abdominis runs vertically on either side of the anterior wall of the abdomen, from the sternum and ribs to the pelvis. There are four sets of two parallel muscle bellies that make up the rectus abdominis and are "separated" by a band of connective tissue called the linea alba (see Figure 3.2). The linea alba is known as the white line. It is white when dissected and collagenous in nature. The linea alba runs vertically from the sternum to the pubic bone, although the fibers themselves tend to run horizontally on ultrasound imaging. The linea alba is the fusion of all aponeuroses of the side muscles of the abdomen.

EXTERNAL OBLIQUES

The external obliques are one of the three sets of muscles on the side of the abdomen, to the side of the rectus abdominis. The muscle fibers of the external obliques run obliquely downward and toward the front of the body in the same direction as if you were putting your hands into your front pockets. The external oblique muscle fibers arise from your lower eight ribs and then form an aponeurosis that passes toward the front and inserts at the midline in the linea alba. This aponeurosis of the external obliques runs on top of the rectus abdominis muscle. The lower aspect of the aponeurosis inserts into the anterior superior iliac crest (a point at the front of the pelvis where you would rest the laundry basket; Figure 3.2) and reaches over to your pubic bone forming the inguinal ligament (the grease/groin where your pelvis meets the leg). The function of the external obliques is trunk flexion and opposite side rotation when working unilaterally with the trunk.

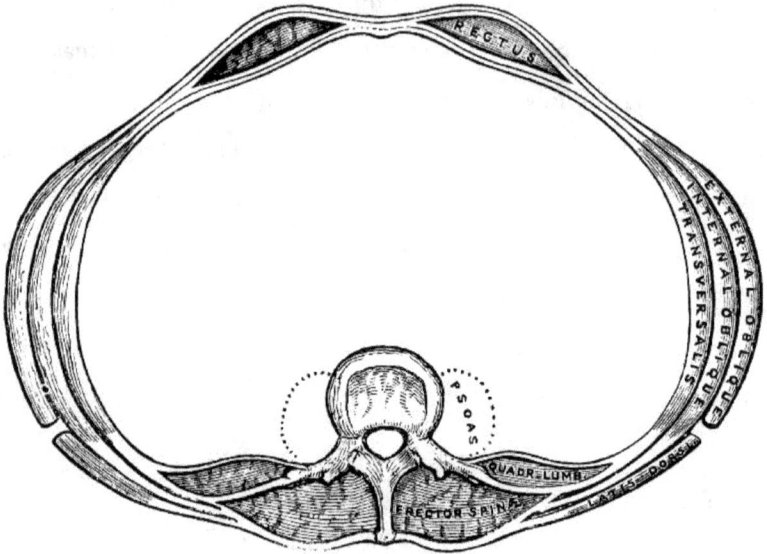

Figure 3.3. Superior view:
fascia of the abdominal muscles.
From Morphart Creation/*Shutterstock.com.*

INTERNAL OBLIQUES

The internal obliques are located below the external obliques and contain the largest mass of muscle bulk of the three muscles on the side of the abdomen. The fibers of the internal obliques run perpendicular to the external obliques. The muscle fibers originate at the ·lumbar fascia, the iliac crest, and the lateral two thirds of the inguinal

LET ME TURN YOU ON

ligament, and then run upward to form another aponeurosis. Above the arcuate line, the aponeurosis bifurcates to encapsulate the rectus abdominis. Below the arcuate line, the aponeurosis only passes anteriorly to the rectus abdominis. The arcuate line is actually a visible line found between the umbilicus and the pubic bone, which is created by the fascial differences at this level — the fascia are thicker above the arcuate line and thinner below.

The function of the internal obliques is flexion of the trunk and lateral flexion and rotation to the same side when working unilaterally. The internal obliques also assist in forced expiration.

PYRAMIDALIS

Not everyone is blessed with the pyramidalis muscle; it is a common abnormality not to have one. In many anatomy books it is not even shown. The pyramidalis muscle is a small set of muscles that lie over the lower portion of the rectus abdominis, just above the pubic bone. It is present in about ninety percent of the population.[1]

WHERE IS THE TRANSVERSE ABDOMINIS?

The transverse abdominis is one of the deep core muscles, located just below the internal obliques (see Figure 3.3). This is the muscle we are most interested in when we discuss strengthening the deep core of the abdomen. The transverse abdominis is the thinnest muscle belly group of the three muscle bellies on the side of your abdomen. It is made up of slightly more Type 1 fibers (slow twitch) and these muscle fibers run horizontally around the abdominals.[2] Slow twitch fibers are long-acting muscles primarily designed for endurance.

The transverse abdominis originates from the lower six costal cartilages of your free ribs, the lumbar fascia, and the iliac crest.[3] The aponeurosis of the transverse abdominis is located below the rectus abdominis, except in the lower two bellies of the rectus abdominis, where it goes above (see Figure 3.4).

WHY IS THE TRANSVERSE ABDOMINIS SO IMPORTANT?

TAKE NOTICE that you have no bones supporting you from your sternum down to your pelvis in the front aspect of your lower torso. This lack of supporting bones means that it is particularly important to strengthen the abdominal muscles, along with the associated tendons and fascia. Together, the fascia, linea alba, and abdominal muscles act as your support system. The lack of bony attachments in your abdomen also emphasizes the importance of muscle and fascia in making significant changes in alignment.

I find changing the physiology of muscle and fascia to be significantly more lasting than bony adjustments for alignment, strength, and the elimination of pain. In fact, strengthening and manipulating muscle and fascia aligns bone. Many people only think about aligning the spine, for example, using the path of bones. These people often rely on frequent chiropractic bony adjustments and many have no real lasting change in their alignment and strength. Simple, quick adjustments in bone are often not permanent, lasting changes in your body. It seems clear to me that muscles are more dynamic and have more potential to align your spine compared to bony adjustments or manipulations. Muscles have memory, they talk, and they have dynamic neurological pathways. "Muscle talk" is a real thing. Plus, you can control your muscles. And muscles move your bones.

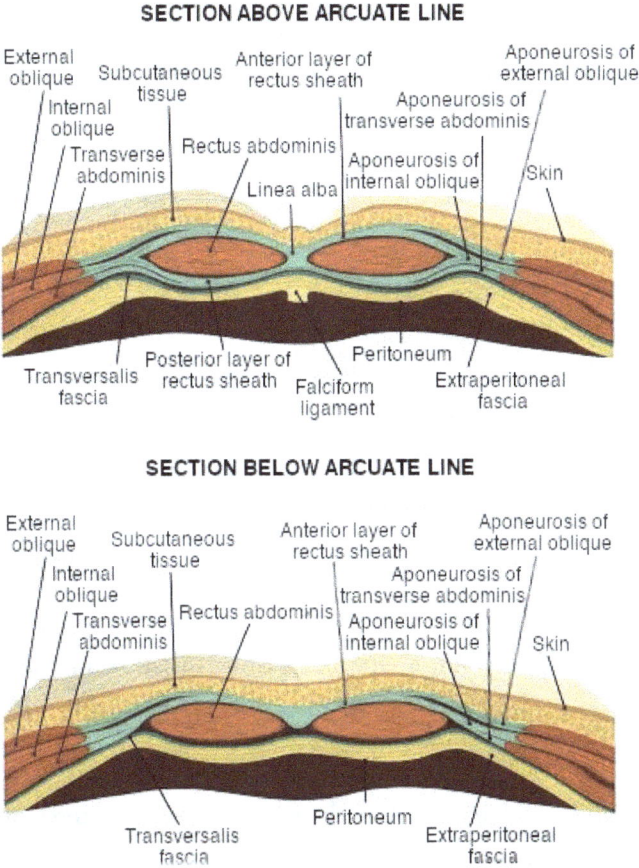

SECTION ABOVE ARCUATE LINE

External oblique | Subcutaneous tissue | Anterior layer of rectus sheath | Aponeurosis of external oblique
Internal oblique
Transverse abdominis | Rectus abdominis | Aponeurosis of transverse abdominis
Linea alba | Aponeurosis of internal oblique | Skin
Transversalis fascia | Posterior layer of rectus sheath | Falciform ligament | Peritoneum | Extraperitoneal fascia

SECTION BELOW ARCUATE LINE

External oblique | Subcutaneous tissue | Anterior layer of rectus sheath | Aponeurosis of external oblique
Internal oblique
Transverse abdominis | Rectus abdominis | Aponeurosis of transverse abdominis | Aponeurosis of internal oblique | Skin
Transversalis fascia | Peritoneum | Extraperitoneal fascia

Figure 3.4. Fascia of the abdominal muscles above and below the arcuate line.
Adapted from Logika600/*Shutterstock.com*.

Note the back and front attachments of the fascia of the transverse abdominis in Figures 3.3 and 3.4. What better corset can you find? See how integrated the transverse abdominis muscle is? In the front, the muscle belly of the transverse abdominis ends at the muscle bellies of the rectus abdominis, but extends itself in the form of an aponeurosis. Looking at the back, the transverse abdominis connects to the thoracolumbar fascia (which branches into the anterior, middle, and posterior layers) and attaches indirectly to your back muscles, psoas (deep-seated hip and core muscle), and lastly to your backbone. The transverse abdominis is a well-connected muscle that has the ability to provide a strong and dynamic built-in corset.

WHILE I SEE THE TRANSVERSE ABDOMINIS, DO YOU?

The individual in Figure 3.5 appears to have a nice display of the transverse abdominis. I say "appears" because true function and strength is best seen in real life, alive, in both static and dynamic positions. Now let me help YOU see it by pointing out a few of the characteristics that I see.

There is tension at the linea alba. This tension will further allow the ability to develop the rectus abdominis muscle. Notice the defined rectus abdominis muscle, outlined by the linea alba in the center of the abdomen and by the start of the aponeuroses from the side muscles of the abdomen. The linea alba, again, is a collagenous tissue tougher than skin or muscle that runs from the xiphoid process (the smallest and most inferior region of the sternum) to the pubic bone. If you do not have tension at the linea alba, most likely the transverse abdominis is weak. Without tension at the linea alba, it is difficult, if not impossible, to develop your rectus abdominis.

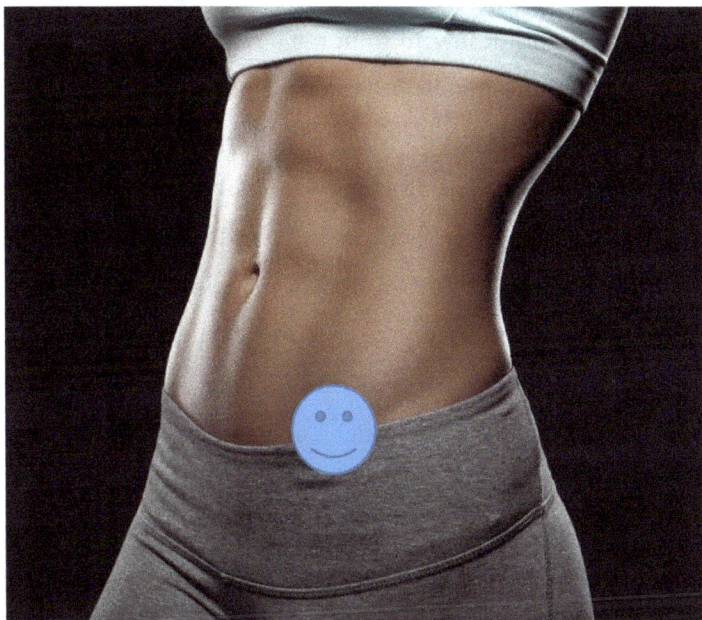

Figure 3.5. View of the transverse abdominis from the outside. The blue smiley face marks the location of notable transverse abdominis muscle bulk. Adapted from Fresh Stock/*Shutterstock.com.*

In Figure 3.5, if you look at the midline from pubic bone to sternum, there is no splitting or thinning of the linea alba. It appears to be sitting together nicely and firmly. The abdominal contents are held snugly and there is no sagging of tissues (fat, skin, muscle, fascia). The skin appears healthy. Clinically, if there is a gap at the linea alba, often the skin will appear aged (saggy, wriggly, discolored, thinned). There is often some bulging of the internal organs and muscle with increased pressure or at rest.

I can see that the transverse abdominis is active. I see tone. It is *turned on* and working for her. The muscle of the transverse abdominis (verses the fascia and tendon of the muscle) has some bulk, most notably seen just inward from the iliac crest and outward from the rectus abdominis muscle bellies (look for the blue smiley face in Figure 3.5). The iliac crest is the bone on the side of the pelvis, commonly used as a stable resting point while carrying a baby or a laundry basket. It is also where backpackers put the attached supporting belt of their backpacks so that it distributes weight correctly over the pelvis and causes less stress on the back and shoulders.

Notice the space between the ribs and the iliac crest. This person does not appear overly tight or guarded. If the abdominal muscles and lower back muscles are too tight, the ribs can actually sit on or in the pelvis. Yes! I have seen and felt it happen. Her ribs do not appear to be out too far, which would look more like a barrel chest. Her ribs do not appear to be in too far. Both of these abnormalities could indicate poor activation and mobility of the transverse abdominis along with other muscles of the lower and mid torso.

IDENTIFY YOUR TRANSVERSE ABDOMINIS

Look and feel specifically at and below the underwear line (see smiley face in Figure 3.5); that is where the bulk of transverse abdominis muscle is best felt and seen on ultrasound imaging. In fact, I tell my patients when their transverse abdominis is weak to get comfortable with their hands in their pants until this muscle is mastered. Specifically, I tell them to palpate (touch) just inward an inch or two from the anterior superior iliac spine of the iliac crest, just below the underwear line (Figure 3.6). When the transverse abdominis muscle is on, it should have some tone and bulk. Again, it is best identified from the iliac crest (specifically inward and down one to two inches from the anterior superior iliac spine of the iliac crest).

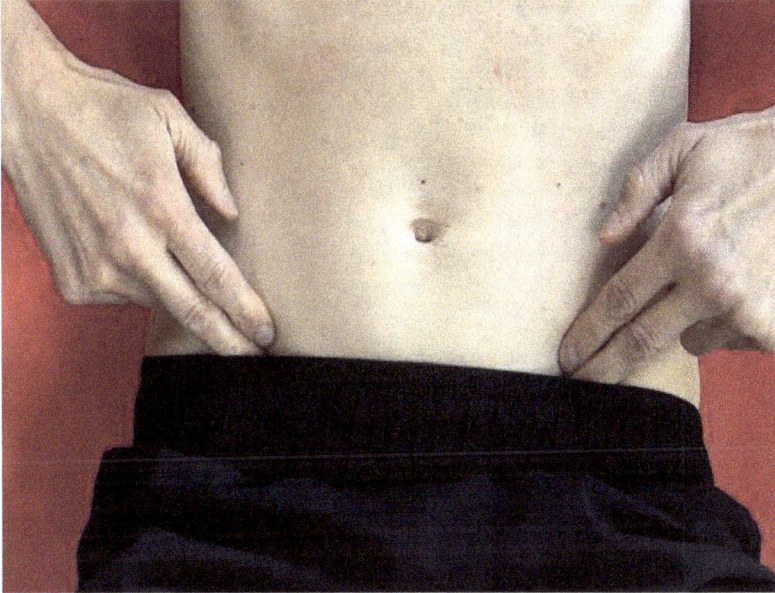

Figure 3.6. To feel the transverse abdominis, palpate just inward from the anterior superior iliac spine of the iliac crest.

For patients who have a weak transverse abdominis, after they have learned how to activate and identify the muscle, I then have them activate their transverse abdominis with their normal activities of daily living until eventually it is on and working automatically. The length of time before the transverse abdominis starts working automatically will be different for everyone and depends on current strength, life, rest, diet, and motivation. Again, to turn these muscles on, you have to think about them as you do all of your daily activities.

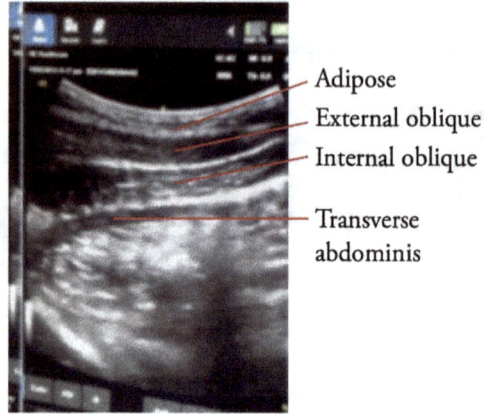

Figure 3.7. An ultrasound image of the side abdominal muscles. From Danny Crawford.

Real time diagnostic ultrasound is another technique used to see the transverse abdominis and other abdominal and pelvic floor muscles. It is a form of biofeedback, a way to gain greater awareness of one's own body. This is something I commonly use in the clinic to assist patients in identifying their transverse abdominis. Imaging also assists in re-training the deep core muscles to work properly. With a diagnostic ultrasound machine, you can compare both sides of the transverse abdominis; it is not uncommon to see distinct differences between sides when working with patients. You can also see co-activation of the pelvic floor along with the transverse abdominis. You can see the muscles in action, including their ability to contract and move or glide. You can also see if compensations are happening at nearby muscles. And, obviously, you can also see the morphology of the muscles. Trained pelvic floor therapists do use ultrasound machines, but they are not commonly seen in most clinics due to the costs involved in investing in such equipment and the training needed to successfully use them.

If we go back to Figure 3.7, the third space from the top of the screen, the thinnest of the muscles, is the transverse abdominis. From the top of the image down, you can first see adipose tissue (which is white), then the external oblique (which is mainly black with some white), then the internal oblique, normally the thickest of the three muscles (which is mainly black with some white), and finally the transverse abdominis. The transverse abdominis does not have a lot of white area, which I hypothesis is because it is an endurance muscle and not made to store fat. White can indicate muscle striations and adipose. Because the transverse abdominis should be *on* to some degree at all times to help support your posture, breath, and stability, I would not suspect adipose to develop.

Clinically, the transverse abdominis muscle continues to appear black on ultrasound imaging even in unconditioned and obese people. Furthermore, I have never seen the transverse abdominis muscle to be bigger than the oblique muscles in bulk. In some surgical patients, especially those with a history of abdominal wounds, I have seen the transverse abdominis muscle severely thinned or even missing in part. The deep core is never, or rarely, discussed after surgery, and unfortunately many do not even know that damage has occurred following surgery.

THE FUNCTIONS OF THE TRANSVERSE ABDOMINIS:
STATIC AND DYNAMIC STABILITY

Static and dynamic stability are the major reasons for learning about, caring for, and maximizing the potential of the transverse abdominis. This muscle is vast, encompassing your entire lower core. This is the basis for your body's stability. This is your dynamic human girdle. Unlike a fabric girdle, this is a fully responsive human girdle, constantly adapting to meet your needs. If it is functioning in a correct manner, then it is *turned on*, to some degree, all of the time. The transverse abdominis is continually assisting with stabilization like two gentle hands holding your lower core and pelvis in place. The transverse abdominis acts like a mother's hand around a child's waist as she is learning to walk for the first time. The muscle provides just enough assistance to stabilize, but not to squeeze the abdominal cavity organs and intestines.

TRY THIS DRILL: Stand on one leg. Now let someone gently hold onto your pelvis as you balance; you should notice a feeling of ease and stability.

There is power in the stability of the lumbopelvic region in both sport and life. This stability allows for power and agility of movement, which makes it crucial to have the transverse abdominis in good working order. Imagine if a sense of ease and stability could be felt with every run, with every weight-bearing phase.

Now, many who try this drill, unfortunately, will feel less

stable. This can happen when the body is compensating for an imbalance somewhere else in the body. In this case, providing stability at the lumbopelvic junction interferes with an individual's current alignment and movement patterns and is not wanted. This person needs physical therapy in order to find the cause of the misalignment and restore normal function of the transverse abdominis. Sometimes, by correcting whatever imbalance exists, the transverse abdominis will naturally fire again. The transverse abdominis needs to be positioned for success, i.e., alignment needs to be corrected. I often assess and restore the transverse abdominis, along with the rest of the deep core, with my patients, if possible.

THE TRANSVERSE ABDOMINIS ASSISTS WITH
URINE AND BOWEL CONTINENCE

When the transverse abdominis muscle is not firing correctly, it can place unnecessary stress on the pelvic floor. The pelvis will not be as stable and connected, because it will not have its natural girdle holding it in place. The pelvic floor will also have to work harder to keep the pelvis together as it fights forces of instability from above.

I feel that the transverse abdominis muscle is equally as important as the pelvic floor in restoring lumbopelvic stability, and that importance extends to restoring or maintaining continence of both bladder and bowel. Studies have not quite proved this, but clinically, if the transverse abdominis is weak along with the pelvic floor, I would argue that these muscles are equally important in maintaining/restoring continence. I have seen many weak pelvic floors with no incontinence, indicating that the pelvic floor is not always the muscle to blame for the leaking of urine. Therefore, strengthening the pelvic floor is often not the cure to incontinence. However, physicians and therapists continue to simply tell patients to do pelvic floor contractions. The transverse abdominis and pelvic floor are both breathing muscles, they are both stabilizing muscles along with the rest of the deep core, and their functions, working together and independently, are important for maintaining continence and stability.

WHAT ELSE DOES THIS MUSCLE DO?

Breathing

The transverse abdominis muscle assists with expanding the abdominal muscles outward during inhalation and inward during exhalation. Forced expiration increases activation of the transverse abdominis. As a breathing muscle, the transverse abdominis helps to create and regulate pressure differentials between the thoracic and abdominal cavities. This affects the dynamics of all fluid systems: blood, lymph, and cerebral spinal fluid. For some patients, abdominal binders are used to restore abdominal pressure and improve breathing capacity.

Dysfunctional breathing (inappropriate breathing which is persistent enough to cause symptoms with or without apparent organic cause) is suspected to be a major cause of primary care provider visits, but currently it is not clearly identified. As a physical therapist focusing on the deep core, I have noticed many diagnoses associated with poor breathing patterns including postural orthostatic tachycardia syndrome (POTS), GERD, bladder incontinence, stomach and back pain, poor digestion, anxiety, etc.

There is a close relationship between normal breathing and normal core functioning. Furthermore, there is a relationship between illness and poor deep core functioning. The transverse abdominis is one of the primary deep core breathing muscles, and often, restoring the function of the traverse abdominis improves medical diagnoses.

Improved Organ Function

Another function of the transverse abdominis is the mobilization of your organs. The transverse abdominis lengthens and shortens as you breathe, creating a rise and fall in internal pressure. Decompressing and compressing. This movement can assist the intestines with digestion. The transverse abdominis is also one of the primary muscles to assist in the evacuation of the bowel. When patients have difficulty having a bowel movement, this is the primary muscle I have them strengthen. This muscle can also be used to improve the flow of urine. The transverse abdominis compresses the bladder and the bowel to assist with the evacuation of waste from the body. Furthermore, it helps to stabilize the lumbopelvic region, taking stress off of the pelvic floor so that it can relax to evacuate bowel and/or bladder.

Prevention and Treatment of Back Pain

The transverse abdominis is able to decrease low back pain and prevent musculoskeletal diagnoses through stability and decompression forces. Let's go back a bit — how does the transverse abdominis muscle help with low back pain? As I have explained in the previous sections, the transverse abdominis is like a dynamic corset or girdle, assisting in stabilizing your pelvis, which is *your foundation*. The transverse abdominis helps to keep the spine protected and aligned. The transverse abdominis is also a breathing muscle and each breath acts as a natural decompression system on your spine. This decompression preserves the spine by relieving load and encouraging blood flow, assisting with prevention and treatment of low back pain.

With each breath, the transverse abdominis has the ability to decompress and compress the abdominals. The amount of eccentric and concentric contracting with the breath will depend on the task that you are doing. People pay big bucks for decompression traction machines, devices, and therapy, but we have a built-in system to improve our spinal health — THE DEEP CORE.

One of my first clinical positions as a student physical therapist was with a specialist of the spine. Every single one of his patients did core stabilization exercises, despite their spinal diagnoses. Core stabilization exercises involve activation and strengthening of the transverse abdominis. These exercises are very effective for multiple spinal diagnoses, acute to chronic, resulting from all types of musculoskeletal diagnoses. The transverse abdominis is the key muscle to focus on to decrease pain in the lumbar spine from musculoskeletal low back pain. Musculoskeletal low back pain is often the diagnosis that is given when no clearly defined issue is found on an X-ray, MRI, or CT scan. I find it odd that pain is a medical diagnosis; in my eyes, pain is a symptom. Furthermore, it is a subjective complaint by the patient. We must ask ourselves, why are we in pain?

The point is that the transverse abdominis muscle has the ability to help with multiple lumbar diagnoses, such as spinal stenosis, spondylosis, spondylolisthesis, degenerative disc disease, herniated discs, and scoliosis. In fact, the transverse abdominis helps with the general health of the whole spine by stabilizing it from unwanted shear, compressive, and tensile forces. If you don't have a stable platform, the rest of the spine will have to compensate.

Some people with quite alarming X-rays and MRIs are living with no pain and no motor and/or sensory loss whatsoever. These are important facts to note. Just because you don't have pain does not mean you don't have a problem. And, even if you have a valid diagnosis and visual evidence on scans, it does not always mean that your pain is from that particular diagnosis.

As a personal example, I have scoliosis. I have what is called a 4C curve of the spine with two curves — one in the lumbar spine and the other in the thoracic. However, I live with no low back pain at all currently. Several experts in the area of the spine have been shocked to see on imaging that I have two near twenty-degree curves of the spine. The scoliosis is not so obvious in part because I focus on activating and strengthening the deep core.

I have shared this to reinforce something for you — imaging is just one moment in time. For this reason, try not to get overly excited about the perceived results of your own imaging or scans. Instead, try to make sure that all of your core muscles are firing and focus on improving and correcting your posture, alignment, and form. Also, find a good physical therapist to help you resolve your individual issues.

Hernias

The abdominal muscles do have some weak spots that you need to pay attention to. These particular spots are common areas for hernias to develop (see Figure 3.8). About ten percent of hernias occur from incisions.[4] A hernia is an abnormal protrusion of abdominal contents through a defect in the abdominal wall. One weak spot is the inguinal region, the inguinal canal; seventy-five percent of hernias occur at the inguinal region (see Figure 3.9).[4] The inguinal canal contains the vas deferens, testicular artery and veins, cremasteric artery, and artery of vas in males and the round ligament in females. In both females and males it contains inferior epigastric vessels, the genitofemoral nerve, and lymphatic vessels.

Chronic hernia without repairs, multiple hernias, multiple hernia repairs, or unsuccessful hernia repairs may make restoration of the transverse abdominis more difficult. It will also be hard to recover the transverse abdominis if the cause of the hernia is still present. Surgery does not always fix the cause, and the hernia will likely return if the cause is still there.

What causes hernias? Congenital defects, loss of tissue strength and elasticity (from aging or repetitive stress), operative trauma, and increased abdominal pressure (from obesity, chronic pulmonary diseases, lifting, ascites, pregnancy, inflammation, tumors) are some of the reasons. In my opinion, another cause would be lack of functional strength and mobility of the transverse abdominis. Excessive extension of the spine and/or tightness of the back and/or abdominal muscles could be another cause.

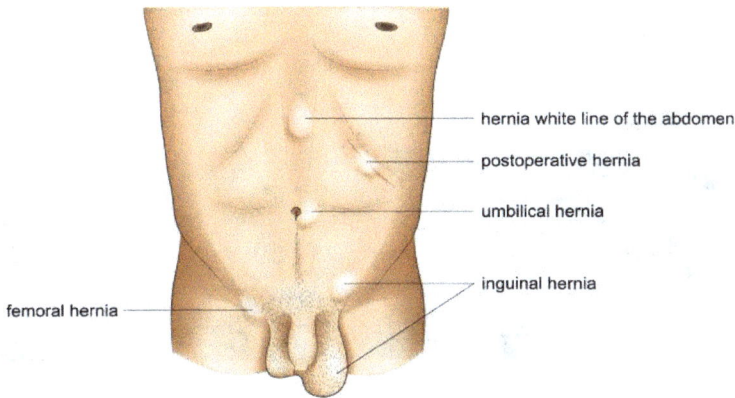

Figure 3.8. Examples of hernias.
From Artemida-psy/*Shutterstock.com.*

It is possible for hernias to cause strangulation of the intestines. If the intestines protrude through the hernia, blood flow can be cut off secondarily, leading to necrosis (tissue death), bowel obstruction, or infection.

As a physical therapist, I think the more common risk with having a hernia is developing a weak core. Pain and the rare strangulation may be possible, but decreased performance and stability are more likely. Hernias are holes in your abdominal tissue; it is nearly impossible to fully develop abdominal muscles around even a small hole. Imagine your bicep without a connection at either end to your shoulder or forearm; how could the muscle push or pull to grow?

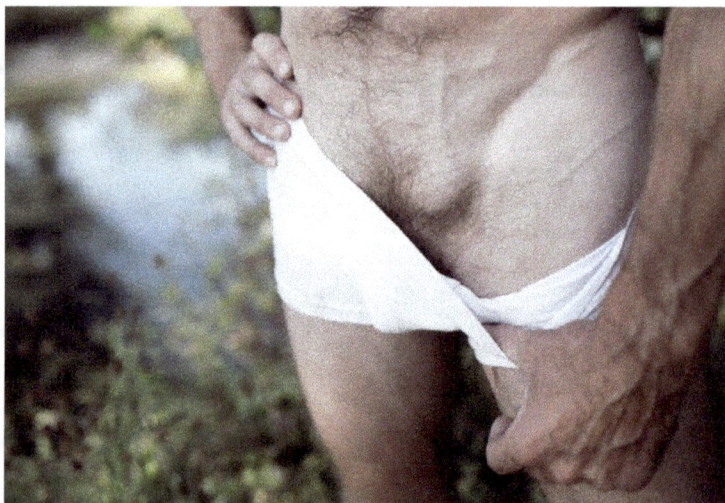

Figure 3.9. An inguinal hernia.
From Skeronov/*Shutterstock.com.*

Hernias cannot be fixed with exercise. Surgery is needed to reconnect the tissues. Without surgical repair, you are at a real risk of the hernia getting bigger and increasing your instability.

Are there any other ways to repair a hernia so the tissues can communicate, reconnect, heal, and strengthen? How else could we connect these tissues that are no longer bound? I have tried taping to assist in drawing the tissue back together. I have also seen others attempt taping without success. Taping can be painful. I also wonder if vacuum-assisted closure technology could help with hernias of the abdomen; this technology is currently used to assist with wound healing following surgery.

Hernia repair involves cutting fascia, and potentially muscle, so it is important to find a good surgeon. You have to ask yourself, "How is the surgeon putting this fascia or muscle back together?" Much like a torn sweater given to a tailor for repair, you have to ask, "Will this sweater ever be the same?" The answer to this question is very important. Find the best surgeon, just as you would find the best tailor for an exceptional suit or dress. Remember that there are multiple fascial and muscle layers. Is the surgeon stitching each layer separately so that they can glide? Glide is important — is your transverse abdominis gliding? Real time ultrasound can reveal this. Will it be gliding after surgery?

DIASTASIS RECTI ABDOMINIS AND LINEA ALBA

As mentioned previously, the linea alba runs from the xiphoid process to the pubic bone and is situated between the left and right rectus abdominis bellies. *Diastasis recti abdominis* is the separation of the rectus abdominis muscles commonly known as the six-pack. This can occur in males and females, but it is common to see this during pregnancy due to the stretching of the fascia and/or connective tissue.

While the fetus grows in the uterus, the linea alba can thin and elongate along the horizontal plane. The horizontal distance between the rectus abdominis musculature is referred to as the inter-recti distance. Rath et al have used inter-recti distances greater than

0.9 centimeter when measured halfway between the pubic bone and the umbilicus, 2.7 centimeters just above the umbilicus, and 1.0 centimeter halfway between the umbilicus and xiphoid as diagnostic criteria for diastasis recti abdominis among individuals below forty-five years of age.[5] Diagnostically, diastasis recti abdominis is anything outside of normal means. Studies have shown increased risk of developing diastasis recti abdominis with pregnancy.[6] The most common site of diastasis recti abdominis is at the umbilicus; left untreated, this has been linked to lumbopelvic pain.[7] Increased weight at the gut can also cause elongation of the linea alba — this is not just a diagnosis in pregnancy. Clinically, I find diastasis recti abdominis diagnoses more common above the umbilicus in males and at or below the umbilicus in females.

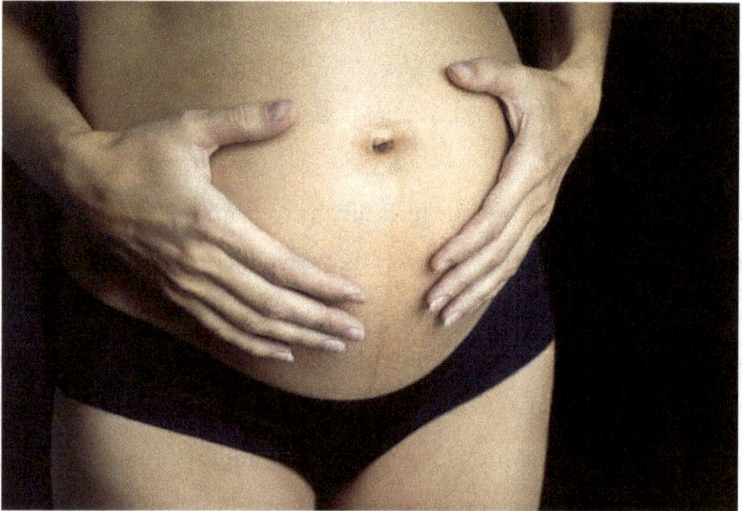

Figure 3.10. Linea nigra. Note the darker pigmentation of skin at midline above underwear and going superior and then into and around the umbilicus.
From Maxim Blinkov/*Shutterstock.com.*

Clinically, I have also noted increased pigment changes at the linea alba where diastasis recti abdominis is identified in females. This pigmentation is called linea nigra, a dark vertical line between the right and left muscle bellies of the rectus abdominis muscles (Figure 3.10). Although I do not know of any research to connect the pigmentation to diastasis recti abdominis, I believe the increased pigmentation is from toxins within the stomach being released through the thinning linea alba tissue. My theory is that toxins are able to exit more easily secondary to the thinning of the linea alba. Often with restoration of the transverse abdominis and improved tension at the linea alba, I have been able to assist with eliminating this hyperpigmentation.

I would argue that the inter-recti distance is less important than the thickness and tone of the linea alba in providing lumbopelvic stability. Tension is needed 1) to provide support for the rectus abdominis to develop muscle mass, 2) for direct support from the pubic bone to the xiphoid process to prevent over extension of the spine and anterior tilt of the pelvis, and 3) to assist in lumbopelvic stability.

Take note of Figure 3.11. This individual has a lack of tension along her midline (linea alba). Her rectus abdominis and transverse abdominis are not developed. Notice how the skin tissue is not toned, active, or firm. It actually appears "older" too. It is wrinkly and saggy. This is lack of flow, stagnation, which leads to aging – SEE? I have seen some really old looking stomach tissue on otherwise young and healthy skin.

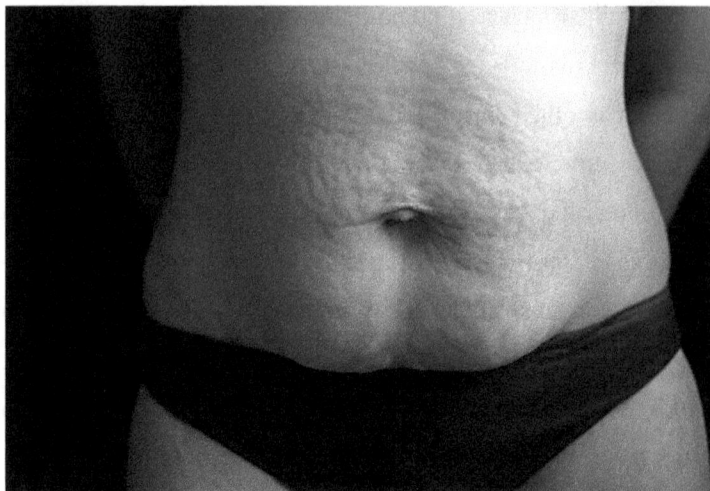

Figure 3.11. Stagnant stomach tissue.
From Elena Khairullina/*Shutterstock.com.*

WHAT DOES ACTIVATION OF THE TRANSVERSE ABDOMINIS DO TO THE INTER-RECTI DISTANCE?

Activating the transverse abdominis does not always shorten the inter-recti distance. In fact, activating the transverse abdominis can actually lengthen this distance. This can be visibly seen and also viewed on ultrasound imaging. On imaging, the horizontal lines of the linea alba often become taut, thicken, and often lengthen, creating tension. Tension allows for stability.

SURGICAL INCISIONS AND YOUR TRANSVERSE ABDOMINIS

In any abdominal surgery, not just a hernia repair, your deep core muscles and/or fascia are being cut and, for some surgeries, removed.

Surgery is a form of trauma to tissue in and of itself, even with the best of surgical options. Is robotic surgery the best for the abdominal muscles? Instead of one larger incision you now have multiple puncture wounds. Imagine taking your shirt to the tailor; would you want multiple tears and repairs or one bigger one? In some cases, I would opt for robotic surgery, as the need for precision will outweigh the number of small incisions received. In other cases, I would opt for one bigger incision to avoid multiple cuts into my tissue.

Again, how are the tissues being put back together? Are the tissues being put back together? With any abdominal surgery, it is important to have a doctor who understands the importance of deep core strength. The ones who understand should be discussing how they are going to preserve your deep core prior to surgery. There are multiple layers of fascia and muscle. These muscles and fascial layers glide over each other, which is important body mechanics. If all layers are stitched all together in a bundle, how can they glide? What if they are not all stitched back together, but rather, the doctors only address some of the layers? How can you restore tension for strength in all of your abdominal layers?

Surgery does not fix strategy. Surgery does not fix all of the musculoskeletal imbalances caused by the need for surgery. One of the ghastliest things I see physicians do after surgery is say, "You don't need therapy." Now this makes NO sense. If you have had a weak, dysfunctional, arthritic hip for five years, and now decide to have surgery, you have been limping and your muscles have compensated for the pain. Furthermore, why is your hip arthritic? Many times, it is an alignment problem. Did surgery fix the muscle-motor memory and pain behaviors, and re-align all the soft tissue (ligament, fascia, muscle, bone)? Did it release all the muscles that are tight from guarding? NO — surgery did not fix strategy. When looking at abdominal surgery, the same issues need to be addressed. Are your abdominal muscles *turned on*, are they aligned? Are they restricted? Are they functional? Is there scar tissue? The trauma of surgery alone is worthy of treating: swelling, scar tissue, fatigue from medication, lack of mobility, to name a few very possible side effects.

One of the most disturbing surgeries I have seen is the transverse rectus abdominis muscle (TRAM) flap surgery. With this surgery, the surgeons are cutting part of the rectus abdominis and the aponeurosis of the transverse abdominis, then taking that flap of tissue and tucking it under the skin of the upper abdomen to use as breast tissue. In most cases, the reason for breast removal and reconstruction is breast cancer. This poor person has already suffered the loss of their breast and is now suffering the loss of their abdominal muscles. Mind you, this is an elective surgery, in that patients are supposedly willing to give up their abdominal muscles for breast tissue. However willingly, is it knowingly? Do the doctors really discuss the potential risks of this surgery? Do the doctors even tell the patient that they are using their deep core muscles? Do the doctors know how vital the abdominal strength, tension, and function are? To me this surgery should be illegal — and maybe it is by now in some facilities. The patients I have seen with this surgery did not understand the importance of their abdominal muscles nor the elective surgery. Did their doctors? Sadly, some of the patients thought this was the more "natural" surgery and were clueless to what they had given up. I am very sad to see this!

What is happening to people after abdominal surgery? Most often, return of the abdominal muscles and their function is not even a topic of concern for either the doctor or the patient. I have seen patients come into the outpatient clinical setting following wound vacuum-assisted closure (VAC) treatment with very delicate tissue. Wound VAC is a machine that is placed over the wound to decrease air pressure and assist with healing. These wounds can be very delicate during care and really can remain a delicate area for the rest of the patient's life. I had one patient with a very thinned out circle approximately three inches in diameter at her linea alba. Her tissues felt like tapping on a three-inch diameter drum that could easily break. She did not have contractile properties of fascia or muscle at this site or around it. These wounds and others following surgeries can leave the transverse abdominis compensated and patients at risk for incontinence, poor breathing patterns, low back pain, digestion issues, etc.

SCAR TISSUE

Abdominal surgery can cause scar tissue to form, which can prevent the transverse abdominis from firing properly. Scar tissue can create adhesions in the muscle, fascia, and connective tissue. Scar tissue can disrupt sensory and motor neurons of fascia and muscle and turn the transverse abdominis off or impair its ability to be fully *turned on* and move with full mobility. Fortunately, hands-on techniques and stretching can decrease scar tissue and improve function and appearance significantly.

INFLAMMATION

Inflammation from surgery can cause problems with the contraction of any muscle, including the transverse abdominis. Think of a swollen sprained ankle. The swelling causes a delay in reaction time, limited mobility, and lack of full strength. Just like a swollen ankle, the swelling needs to go down in the abdomen for the muscles to respond with full potential. Rest and ice can be very effective, as well as avoiding activities that increase stress at the lower abdomen. Added inflammation means added recovery time. Stresses that might increase inflammation at the abdominals can include prolonged movement, prolonged sitting or standing, heavy lifting, decreased rest, inflammatory diet, etc.

INTESTINAL INFLAMMATION

Often times intestinal inflammation is the cause of abdominal inflammation and the reason the transverse abdominis muscle is not *turned on*. Conditions like bloating, irritable bowel syndrome, constipation, etc., can cause the intestines to inflame. Inflammatory conditions in the gut should be dealt with by a firm diet focusing on decreasing inflammation, restoring healthy flora, and restoring the gut at a cellular level. It is best to see a licensed dietician and integrative medicine doctor with a focus on diet to restore health and wellness. In cases involving intestinal problems, a change in diet can be quite effective in assisting the transverse abdominis. Physical therapy can also be effective in decreasing inflammation at the gut by correcting any muscular, fascial, and visceral restrictions at the abdomen. Eliminating or decreasing fascial restrictions allows the body to cleanse itself in many physiological ways.

OTHER REASONS THE TRANSVERSE ABDOMINIS IS NOT *TURNED ON*

Pain

The transverse abdominis might not want to *turn on* due to pain. Sometimes activating the transverse abdominis can cause pain at the region of the transverse abdominis or elsewhere. Often contracting the transverse abdominis can cause pain in the lower back or abdominals when there are musculoskeletal imbalances. For example, if the back is too tight (in the fascia, muscle, and bone) or imbalanced, it is possible that the increased force of the transverse abdominis being activated can amplify these imbalances and cause pain. In these cases, it is helpful to improve mobility in the spine before retraining the transverse abdominis.

Peculiarly, activation of the transverse abdominis muscle might cause headache pain. This is something I see more and more. Patients will say, "When I contract the pelvic floor or transverse abdominis, I get a headache." Many professionals will think they are crazy, but bear in mind that the pelvis and sacrum (part of your spine) are connected to the skull via the spinal cord and tissue that backs up the spinal cord. Often when I release the hip and/or pelvic region, I will get a simultaneous release in the neck and vice versa.

However, *more often than not* activating the transverse abdominis muscle assists with decreasing the compression and pain at the
lower back. The transverse abdominis muscle is known to stabilize
and support the back. Like a well-rooted tree, this support reaches
from bottom to top, to the skull. Often strengthening the base of
support — the pelvic floor and transverse abdominis — actually can
and does assist with alleviating headache and neck pain.

Poor Hip Flexor Mechanics

Yet another reason why the transverse abdominis will not want to
turn on is if the hip flexors are doing its job. The stability for the lower core is now coming from the hip muscles instead of the deep core.
This often happens with individuals who have desk jobs or with cyclists who do not cross train or stretch their hip flexors. The hip flexors shorten from sitting or standing slightly bent over. When these
people go to stand up, the hip flexors pull on the front of the spine
and take the spine and hip out of alignment. When the spine is not
aligned, it makes it harder for the deep core to activate.

One can see the importance of getting the hips mobile and
loose in order to not restrict the deep core. Similarly, as previously
discussed, having the ribs and the shoulders loose also helps in not
restricting the core. The same situation can happen with the lower
extremities, the hip flexors being a common cause of poor transverse
abdominis activation. Please note that I use "hip flexors" casually to
refer to the region of the hip flexors and associated structures. For
example, the arteries and nerves, including the femoral nerve, as well

as the fascia involved in the front of the body from the upper leg to the lower spine can shorten.

Abdominal Tightness

Many times the obliques, the rectus abdominis, and the long muscles of the spine will be too tight and limit the ability and/or need of the transverse abdominis to be active and on. Keeping the big abdominal muscles (the obliques and rectus abdominis) consistently tight is like wearing an abdominal brace for too long. The transverse abdominis will turn off or get weak as the brace is taking its job. If this goes on for too long, the transverse abdominis might turn off for good — although this is fixable, as you are learning in this book. Keeping the abdominal muscles tight also affects breathing, as it will be harder to expand the lower intercostal muscles, transverse abdominis, and diaphragm. The body will find a different route, a path of less resistance.

Some people think I am complimenting them when I tell them they have tight abdominal muscles. Unfortunately, this can be quite the contrary. When the rectus abdominis and obliques are at rest, the transverse abdominis should be seen and felt as a breathing muscle. When the rectus abdominis and oblique muscles are too tight, they can restrict breathing. These muscles can also restrict digestion, as well as mobility in the spine and pelvis, and, indirectly, in the extremities. Furthermore, asymmetrical tightness can cause asymmetry of the spine and pelvis.

How do you know if the transverse abdominis is *turned on?* Start to look for the things I have pointed out. Do you have *muscle bulk?* Can you feel the muscle belly below your underwear line? Is your abdomen *coiling and recoiling* when you breathe? Is there *tension at your linea alba?* Are you able to *develop an eight-pack?* Are you free of abdominal *hernias?* Are your *hip flexors loose and not restricting alignment and function of the transverse abdominis?* The long muscles of the hips, arms, and spine are also capable of limiting the strength of the transverse abdominis. Are you able to *empty your bowel and bladder easily?* Are you *continent of urine and bowel?* If you answered "yes" to these questions, then these are all signs that your transverse abdominis is *turned on.*

Are you free of *low back, hip, and pelvic pain and/or achiness?* The cause of low back, hip, and pelvic pain is often a *weak deep core;* the multifidi and transverse abdominis may be weak, therefore putting increased stress on the joints, leading to inflammation, pain, and spinal diagnoses. Or, there may be trigger points and other *soft tissue limitations in your abdominals or back* that are causing low back pain and potentially restricting the function of your transverse abdominis.

HOW DO YOU KNOW IF
THE TRANSVERSE ABDOMINIS IS *TURNED OFF?*

If you answered "no" to any of the previous questions, those are potential signs that you are turned off or not fully *turned on*. Some medical diagnoses that I have seen clinically linked to a weak transverse abdominis include GERD, constipation, bloating, IBS, low back pain, scoliosis, diagnoses related to musculoskeletal alignment, hernias, degenerative disc disease, pregnancy, history of pregnancy, obesity, and incontinence.

ARE YOU STUCK IN AN "ON" POSITION?
NOT COILING AND RECOILING?

If stuck in an "on" position, the transverse abdominis is *turned on* and contracted, but not functioning dynamically. The muscle fibers may be shortened or lengthened or somewhere in between, as the transverse abdominis is stuck in one position or in a restricted position. This can happen when overworking the transverse abdominis muscle or consciously or unconsciously keeping the muscle contracted. The transverse abdominis may want to stay in a limited position due to musculoskeletal imbalances. Whatever the reason, the transverse abdominis may no longer be able to function at all ranges. Just like a frozen shoulder, this lack of range of motion at all planes is considered a weakness. *Mobility is strength.*

Restricted muscles can be seen and felt by experienced hands and eyes. If the transverse abdominis is not coiling and recoiling, one will not see full expansion and contraction of the abdominal musculature and/or ribs. Restrictions may be associated with trigger points, taut bands, fascial restrictions, scar tissue, cysts, masses, adhesions, edema, surgical implants, and even external forces (such as wearing tight pants or energy fields).

Overly tight abdominal musculature is associated with anxiety and breathing problems. Lack of mobility of the transverse abdominis, in particular, might lead to constipation and GERD symptoms or lack of mobility in the back.

TEST YOUR TRANSVERSE ABDOMINIS: ARE YOU *TURNED ON?*

Do You Have Tension at Your Linea Alba?

Note that your linea alba runs from your pubic bone to your xiphoid process (see Figure 3.2). Start by lying flat on your back with your knees bent and feet flat on the floor. Place your fingers on your belly button and gently apply pressure towards your spine.

You are simply feeling for confirmation of tension at midline between the bellies of your rectus abdominis. Start at your belly button and make your way to your pubic bone. Then again start at your belly button and repeat, applying gentle pressure towards your spine but working upwards toward your xiphoid process (the bone at the end of your sternum/chest).

Now lift your head and repeat the same steps above. You should feel no pain. Feel for tension and space between the left and right muscle bellies of your rectus abdominis. The space should feel firm; you should not feel a soft feeling under your fingers (like you are entering your abdominal content). The space between the muscle bellies of the rectus abdominis should be no bigger than two centimeters. If the space is less than two centimeters but NOT firm, this is also of concern.

Remember that TENSION is what you need for support. Tension at the linea alba is increased when the transverse abdominis is activated. This is also how to test for the diagnosis of diastasis recti abdominis.

Breathing Test

Are you breathing with your transverse abdominis? If the transverse abdominis is *turned on* and mobile, you will see movement in the abdominal wall when breathing. With exhalation, you should be able to see the lower abdominals drawing slightly up towards your head, in towards your spine, and together towards midline. With inhalation you should see the abdominals extend outward. Palpation of the transverse abdominis should be done to confirm it is activating with the breath.

Stabilization Test:
Single Straight Leg Raise and Double Straight Leg Raise

Can you stabilize your core while moving your legs? Find a firm surface, the floor would be ideal. Lie flat on your back with your face up. Keep both legs extended to full length. Place your arms flat at your sides, palms up and relaxed, not pushing into the floor with any pressure from shoulder to fingertips. Attempt not to let your lower back come off of the firm surface as you lift one of your legs straight up to about forty degrees. When the lumbopelvic junction is not stable, you will often see a notable shift of the pelvis. The pelvis may shift up or down, side to side, and/or rotate. These are all potential signs of weakness or poor neuromuscular coordination of the transverse abdominis. Again, palpation of the transverse abdominis should be done to confirm findings.

Another sign of weakness of the transverse abdominis with this test would be bulging of the abdominals, usually at midline. The muscles might be stretched, thinned, and unable to hold the abdominal organs and tissues taught. Bulging could also be a sign of over recruitment of the rectus abdominis. Bulges on the sides of the abdomen indicate overuse of the obliques. Bulging anywhere over the abdominals between the ribs and pelvis could also indicate a hernia. Bulging is a sign that the transverse abdominis is not functioning to its full potential or at all.

Excessive arching of the back — over recruitment of the erector spinae — is another sign of a weak transverse abdominis that may be seen with this test. It is not uncommon to see weakness of the transverse abdominis carry over to the multifidi of the deep back muscles, as you will learn in the next chapter.

If the single straight leg raise test is too easy, in that you are able to lift the leg with no signs of weakness, attempt the double straight leg raise. Get into the same position as before. Instead of lifting just one leg to forty degrees, lift both legs up to forty degrees. This is more work for the transverse abdominis, as the weight has doubled. Furthermore, no legs remain on the firm surface to assist with stabilizing. A sign of a weak transverse abdominis will be arching of the lower back. Other signs of weakness with the double leg raise are the same as with the single leg raise.

NOTE: The majority of the population does not have enough lower core strength to do the double leg lift test with good form. This test is *also* a deep core strengthening *exercise* that is often done improperly. It is an *advanced* deep core exercise when done properly.

While lifting the legs in either the single straight leg raise test or the double straight leg raise test, ask yourself "Do I feel my lower abdominals working?" People often compensate by using their back and hip flexors to stabilize and the lower core is not even felt or firing. Make sure when testing and exercising the deep core that you are actually using it. Are you feeling the transverse abdominis contract? Are you feeling the transverse abdominis fatigue? Are you feeling anything in your lower abdominals?

If you are strong in your lower abdominals and transverse abdominis, you might not feel the muscle fatigue. If this is the case, you should also note that it is easy and effortless to keep your back flat; your lower lumbar should not go further into extension (arching). You should also note that your pelvis is not shifting. You should be able to feel the transverse abdominis contract both by touch and in thought. Remember, the transverse abdominis is best felt by placing both hands on your front anterior superior iliac spines and moving your finger inward an inch towards your midline.

Single Leg Transverse Abdominis Test
with Knee and Hip at Ninety–Ninety Position

This test is similar to the single and double straight leg raise tests, however, the knees are bent. Start by lying on your back on a firm, flat surface, ideally the floor. Then bend both of your knees and place your feet flat on the floor. This position is known as "hook-lying". In this position, keep your lower back flat and lift one leg. Keep the knee bent to ninety degrees and make a hip–trunk angle of ninety degrees. Try to keep your lower back from lifting off of the stable surface. Also, attempt to keep your pelvis from moving. This test is not as difficult as the double leg lift, because the weight of the leg is closer to your core and therefore it should be easier to maintain a neutral spine.

If you are unable to keep the lower back from lifting off of the stable surface, this is a sign of a weak transverse abdominis. Similarly, any shift or rotation in the pelvis is a sign of weakness. Any bulge at midline can be a sign of weakness and/or over recruitment of the rectus abdominis muscle. As with the above straight leg raise tests, hernias might prevail with this test.

Common signs of compensation with this exercise include gluteal and hip flexor musculature over activation or hamstring and calf musculature over activation on the leg that is not lifted. Another sign of weakness is extension noted posteriorly at mid thoracic and/ or lumbar spine; patients will come out of neutral spinal alignment.

Double Leg Ninety–Ninety Transverse Abdominis Test

Following the single leg transverse abdominis test with knee and hip at ninety–ninety position, try lifting both legs. After lifting one leg with the knee bent, then lift the other. I like to do this test by lifting one leg at a time to the ninety–ninety position rather than simultaneously lifting both legs. This test is harder than lifting a single leg as no support remains on the stable surface. If you are unable to do this test, this is a sign that your transverse abdominis is weak. I would not classify the transverse abdominis as being weak if the double *straight* leg raise is failed; however, I do believe the transverse abdominis is functionally too weak if unable to do the double leg ninety–ninety test. If an individual is able to do the double straight leg raise test correctly, I would classify them as having a strong deep transverse abdominis.

Linea Nigra Can Be An Indication of Weakness

The linea nigra, as noted previously, is a dark line on the midline of the abdominals between the right and left rectus abdominis muscle bellies seen during and/or after pregnancy. Interestingly, when the transverse abdominis muscle is strengthened and tension is restored at the midline, this line tends to disappear. I have not had one case where it has not. So the presence of linea nigra is one way I check to see if there is some weakness at the linea alba and transverse abdominis following and/or during pregnancies.

Who Is Dominating Your Abdominals?
Infrasternal Angle

The infrasternal angle is the angle below the sternum that is made from the ribs on either side (Figure 3.12). If the angle is less than ninety degrees, it is a sign of overuse/recruitment of the internal obliques. The internal obliques assist with exhaling. It can also be a sign that the diaphragm has overly ascended up into the rib cage towards the head.

If the infrasternal angle is larger than ninety degrees, it can be a sign of overuse/recruitment of the external obliques. This could also be an indication that the diaphragm has descended caudally towards the pelvis. A ninety-degree angle at the lower ribs is considered ideal.

It is important to note that if the obliques are being over recruited, often times the transverse abdominis will be weak. In order to measure the infrasternal angle, place the tips of your thumbs at your xiphoid process and the length of your thumbs just under your ribs.

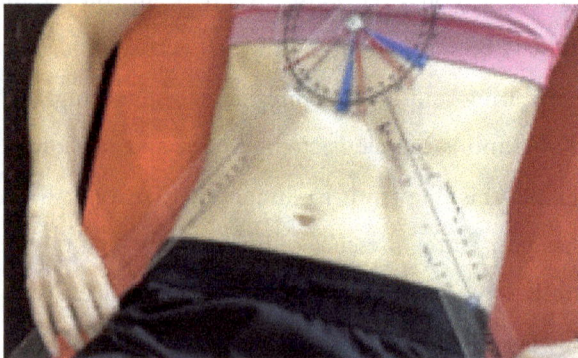

Figure 3.12. Infrasternal angle.

When the transverse abdominis is not firing, you want to learn to identify and isolate it. If you are unable to isolate it, it is acceptable to include other abdominal muscles to get the transverse abdominis started. You can also do certain functional movements that encourage the transverse abdominis to activate. There is some debate among physical therapists regarding whether or not you need to isolate the transverse abdominis. We are going to focus on isolation and identification so YOU KNOW you are *turned on*.

CUEING EXERCISES TO GET

THE TRANSVERSE ABDOMINIS *TURNED ON*

Remember, *cueing* is a verbal command used to get the muscles to do what you want them to do. *These cues are verbal commands to both turn on the transverse abdominis muscle and to strengthen it if it is already on.* Cues may be said aloud or silently within your mind. Cuing involves visualization of the spoken words and then action of the muscle, in this case the transverse abdominis.

Some cues may work for you while others might not have any significance for your brain-to-body connection. Try the following cues to both activate and strengthen your transverse abdominis in isolation:

- Bring hip bones together lightly.
- Bring pelvic bones (anterior superior iliac spine) together.
- With one finger on either side of your belly button (or wherever the weakest point of your abdomen is), lightly bring fingers together.

- With one finger on either side of your belly button (or wherever your weakest point is), imagine bringing your fingers gently apart, as if they were wrapping around the sides of your body to the spine.

LOSE SOME INCHES

When the transverse abdominis muscle has been off and is *turned on*, it can be just a few weeks before my patients begin to notice that their pants are fitting better. When they learn how to turn the transverse abdominis on, it acts as a human girdle and can take inches off the waist. Furthermore, it can assist significantly with low back pain, specifically the achy, daily low back pain that increases with prolonged sitting or standing.

LET'S TURN YOUR TRANSVERSE ABDOMINIS ON: POSITIONING FOR SUCCESS AND NATURAL PROGRESSION

One can use these cues from multiple positions. I like to start in hook-lying position, on the back with the knees bent and the feet on a stable surface. Then I like to progress to side-lying, prone, sitting, standing, walking, squatting, and patient-specific daily tasks. This is the same progression I would use for the pelvic floor muscles, as noted in the previous chapter. Again, the hook-lying position is good because gravity is taken out of the picture. Furthermore, when the knees are bent, the spine is able to get into a more neutral position without the influence of common hip and pelvis restrictions. If you have thoracic and cervical restrictions (upper back and neck), this position will assist in preventing further restrictions. Sometimes placing a pillow under the upper back and/or neck to keep the patient in their current "neutral spine" is also needed for common forward head and shoulder abnormalities seen with desk jobs.

TAKE OUT THE BREATH TO GET STARTED

Taking out the breath is another way to assist in identifying and focusing on the transverse abdominis. Take a breath in, exhale half of the air out, and hold your breath. Then do one of the cues for transverse abdominis activation. When you take out the breath, the body has fewer dynamics to coordinate. This is especially helpful if you are having trouble feeling the transverse abdominis. Many people naturally stop breathing when learning a new skill — remember to progress back to breathing with these exercises and with life.

When first learning, it is ok to do mass practice for a few sets, days, or sometimes weeks without adding the breath to the activation/cuing exercises. Neuromuscular coordination activities and exercises can be exhausting for the mind and body; especially when breathing mechanics are being changed and challenged. Remember that all deep core muscles are also breathing muscles, so every time you are challenging these muscles you are potentially changing your mechanics of breathing.

THINK LIGHT

Do not expect a strong feeling when activating the transverse abdominis. Don't anticipate a big contraction or movement. Think light
and sneaky. For example, "sneak your pelvic bones together." Or
"lightly bring your two fingers on each side of you belly button together with your deepest felt abdominal muscle." Remember this is a
thin, expansive muscle. You might feel the contraction as being light
and insignificant, potentially even a waste of time. Rest assured, it is
not.

FEEL FOR IT

Identify the transverse abdominis through feeling. Feel for tension at
your linea alba with your fingers. Also feel for tension and muscle
contraction directly at the muscle belly. Again, the transverse abdominis muscle bellies are just inward from the anterior superior iliac
spines and below your underwear line. This is where the greatest
muscle bulk of the transverse abdominis is felt.

CO-CONTRACTING TO ACTIVATE
THE TRANSVERSE ABDOMINIS

Remember that the transverse abdominis and the pelvic floor co-contract, meaning they contract together. This is another way to get the
transverse abdominis *turned on* — especially if you are having trouble
isolating or identifying the muscle.

While contracting the pelvic floor, feel for a light contraction in the abdomen; it might seem like nothing, a very light contraction deep in the abdominals. That is the transverse abdominis. Again, it is not a strong feeling when felt in isolation from the other abdominal muscles (rectus abdominis and obliques). Furthermore, the contraction felt by indirectly identifying the transverse abdominis through activation of the pelvic floor is not as strong as when the focus is on the transverse abdominis in a healthy deep core. Intention matters!

One needs to be confident in their ability to isolate the pelvic floor contraction to use this technique as a way to identify and/or *turn on* the transverse abdominis. There is room for error here — for example, if you are contracting all of your abdominal muscles with the pelvic floor contraction then this will not assist in identifying the transverse abdominis. Often it does work though, and can be verified on ultrasound imaging. Another way to verify if correctly identifying and activating the transverse abdominis is to have an experienced physical therapist with good palpation skills assess.

ACTIVATE THE TRANSVERSE ABDOMINIS
WITH A BREATHING CUE

What are the normal mechanics of breathing? A few years ago I was trying to answer this question and figure out what would be considered healthy for the body movements of breathing. I wanted to look at a healthy subject not exposed to societal norms. Societal norms require sitting in church, school, work, and at home for prolonged periods of time. Many adults and children in America have developed poor breathing patterns as we are constantly told to sit still, don't move, stop moving, etc. Often one stops breathing properly with strict cues like "sit still."

We are not meant to sit for six to eight hours at a computer, iPhone, iPad, desk, etc. Doing so can interfere with our deep core mechanics. Many children have developed abnormal movements at very young ages. Since my then four-year-old son had not been sitting still for seven full hours during a school day, I decided to assess the state of his body mechanics used for breathing. What I discovered was that his skin actually moved up, along with the transverse abdominis, and this visible movement was felt below the skin and on top of the fascia. The pressure can actually be seen and felt moving up with exhalation. Following this observation, I decided to add my cuing for the transverse abdominis to the actions of the skin.

Cue for the Transverse Abdominis (One of My Favorites)

Inhale, and then exhale. While exhaling, imagine you are making a light ripple along the skin, like a small wave when a pebble is thrown into the water. Direct the ripple (just under the skin and above your abdominal muscles) from the pubic bone up to your lower ribs and sternum. Stay on top of the water and do not squeeze the abdomen as this may cause pressure to go down to the pelvic floor and increase the risk of prolapse or incontinence. Start by lying down when doing this exercise. Later progress to gravity-dependent positions such as sitting, standing, walking, or running.

HOW TO STRENGTHEN THE TRANSVERSE ABDOMINIS
ONCE IT IS *TURNED ON*

First make sure you can *turn on* the transverse abdominis with the above tests and cues. Then get your baseline. Just like the pelvic floor muscles, determine the endurance of the transverse abdominis muscle. How long can you hold the transverse abdominis contraction before it fatigues or weakens greater than fifty percent? I like to start with this number, and then do ten repetitions of the transverse abdominis contractions six times a day. For example, say you can hold a contraction of the transverse abdominis for five seconds while lying down and then the muscle fatigues greater than fifty percent. Then you would do five-second holds times ten repetitions, six times a day.

You might be asking how you will know when you have fatigued fifty percent. You can assess the amount of fatigue by feeling the contraction with your fingers or kinesthetically. When you let go of the contraction, was there anything to let go of? If you felt no change or movement, then you fatigued one hundred percent before you let go. Or you might notice you lost a percentage of the strength you were originally able to hold or feel when you contracted your transverse abdominis. It is like lifting a weight with a bicep curl; when you start to fatigue it is harder to get to end ranges without poor form (compensations). For the transverse abdominis, activation is lost when the amount of contractile strength is lessened or stopped.

Next you can assess what positions you are able to do the transverse abdominis contractions in. If you can easily do thirty-second contractions while lying down, that's too easy. Make the position harder by adding gravity, body weight, or momentum. Try to do thirty-second contractions of the transverse abdominis while sitting. If you can only hold the transverse abdominis contraction for seven seconds while sitting, and then it fatigues greater than fifty percent, then start with seven-second holds and four seconds of relaxation in sitting. Do six sets of ten a day for mass practice — for results.

IN GENERAL: PROGRESSING THE TRANSVERSE ABDOMINIS WITH POSITIONING

Work your way through this positional progression of transverse abdominis strengthening:

- Take your breath out of the biomechanics. You can take out your breath to assist in identifying and initiating the coordination of the deep core. When you take out the breath, it quiets movement throughout the body and you can better "feel" the transverse abdominis. Obviously you need to breathe and incorporate the breath back into the exercises when you can easily identify the transverse abdominis.
- Gravity is harder than no gravity (lying on the back, stomach, or sides). Gravity can act as a weight and make activation of the transverse abdominis harder. Furthermore, gravity tends to add to poor mechanics that might already exist in the body, making it harder for the deep core to activate. Get into horizontal positions, such as lying on the back, stomach, or sides. In these positions, parts of the body are supported by the floor or ground. Remember, the trans-

verse abdominis muscle and all of the deep core muscles also work to stabilize the body, so take that job away while re-activating or isolating the transverse abdominis by providing the body with a stable surface to rest on. These positions take the weight of the upper body off of the lower core.

- When able to do deep core exercises in horizontal positions, it is time to progress to more vertical positions. Vertical positions stack your body weight and tend to make activation of the transverse abdominis more difficult.

- Sitting is normally harder than lying down because you have added both gravity and your own weight on top of your pelvis. You also add and potentially compound more musculoskeletal issues.

- Standing is harder than sitting because now you have no surface to sit on; the surface can act as an assistant to the pelvic floor and transverse abdominis in their job of supporting the pelvis (until the pelvic floor and transverse abdominis fail from prolonged sitting). Furthermore, imbalances from the lower extremities can now change the dynamics of the pelvis and lumbar region and areas further up the chain.

- Weight is harder than no weight.

- Dynamic positions are harder than stable positions.

- Walking is harder than standing because it requires multiple movements within the body and environment.

- Running is more dynamic than walking — forces are greater and imbalances within the body and environment can also be greater.

Remember, misalignment and posture also impact the ability

of the transverse abdominis to fire. Poor alignment makes activation of the deep core muscles more difficult. The deep core fires best when the spine is aligned; multiple musculoskeletal imbalances at the torso and extremities can change the spinal myofascial and bony alignment.

Also, keep in mind — the above list is a *general list* of progression. There are cases where, for example, individuals can fire the deep core in the most progressive position listed, yet not while lying down.

TRAINING AGAINST GRAVITY

The transverse abdominis needs to be able to fight the forces of gravity in order to be functional. The transverse abdominis is not functional simply because you are able to contract it while lying down. This applies to all of the deep core muscles. A muscle can only hold what it is trained to hold. If you only train the muscle in a state of lying down, it will potentially only work in that position. Remember this when rehabbing a weak or non-functioning deep core. Lying down is especially easy because you do not have to fight gravity.

MAKE IT A LIFESTYLE

The transverse abdominis muscle, like all the core muscles, needs to work for you all day long. So you need to train it all day long. Add the transverse abdominis to your transfers, going from sitting to standing and standing to sitting, for example. Add it to your squats, add it to your breath, and add it to your sport and/or job duties. How easy is it to freely move your extremities while also holding your core in an optimum position? When operating correctly, the deep core should turn on automatically, much like a light bulb does when you walk into a motion-sensor operated room. The transverse abdominis actually contracts prior to movement occurring in the extremities. One should not have to think about the transverse abdominis; it is supposed to be an unconscious response.

You should feel your deep core activate with upper and lower extremity movements. Test yourself: when you lift your arm up, do you feel activation of your transverse abdominis just prior to and throughout the movement? Are you able to hold your pelvis stable when engaged in activities such as running, swimming, or biking? Is your transverse abdominis *on* with these activities? If not, you need to train it to be.

ANOTHER WAY TO STRENGTHEN
THE TRANSVERSE ABDOMINIS: BREATH

Your transverse abdominis muscle is a breathing muscle, assisting you with inhalation and exhalation. Breathing is another way to strengthen this muscle. I like to use the transverse abdominis with exhalation. Focus on full exhalation. Use the transverse abdominis and pelvic floor to force all of the air out of your lungs. When you think you have exhaled all the air, use the transverse abdominis a little more to push any extra air out of the lungs. You can also add an isometric contraction at end range exhalation.

Again, SEX is a great way to have fun while turning on the pelvic floor and transverse abdominis muscles. I strongly recommend sex and masturbation as compliance and consistency are better, both of which give you the results needed to get turned on and to turn on others. Follow the cueing exercises, now with a toy or a partner. You can actually do sets of contractions while masturbating or having intercourse. Or you can just enjoy and see how your hard work has been paying off. Sexual activity can also be used to assist in turning on your transverse abdominis and pelvic floor muscles if they are off. It all depends on where you are with the strength of your pelvic floor and transverse abdominis and what sex is going to do muscularly for you.

ADDING WEIGHT TO THE TRANSVERSE ABDOMINIS

Once you have learned to activate the transverse abdominis and hold isometric contractions in multiple positions, now you can add weight. The weight can start with your own legs or arms. For example, the single leg transverse abdominis test with knee and hip at ninety–ninety can also strengthen the transverse abdominis. Repeat the leg lift ten times, six times a day. When that becomes easy, you can progress to double leg lifts.

Another way to progress is by moving the leg, which is like adding weight for your core. Simply start to straighten your leg a little further each time when lifting.

Another way to add weight is to literally use a resistance band or weights while activating the transverse abdominis. Simply lifting weights with your arms while activating the transverse abdominis is, in essence, adding weight for your transverse abdominis and strengthening it. So, contract the transverse abdominis muscle while lifting weights, squatting, deadlifting, etc. It should naturally be on during these activities, but if you have been turned off or weak for a long time, you will have to retrain the transverse abdominis to work for you. There might be certain segments of the transverse abdominis that are weak; make sure to monitor the weak segments as you add weight.

DON'T FORGET YOUR POSTURE

Position is key when activating the deep core. We should aim for a neutral spine; however, many people cannot get into neutral spinal alignment. There are often too many layers of misaligned tissue (bone, muscle, fascia, connective tissue) that do not allow for full mobility and therefore a neutral spine. In this case, you have to put yourself into a position where your deep core can fire. This is your current "neutral" spine, as close as you can get it to neutral while supporting your current restrictions.

With a neutral lumbopelvic junction, both your multifidi and transverse abdominis should be able to activate. If your hip flexors are tight, you cannot lie "straight" on your back as this will pull you out of getting to a neutral spine position. The tight hips will cause lumbar overextension making it harder to activate the deep core. Thus, train in a position where you are on slack, not pulled to your end range. Start in a supine position (lying on your back) with your knees bent. You might also have to prop your head up to compensate for a classical forward head position. Support your musculoskeletal imbalances, and with time the deep core will assist in aligning you better, BUT the deep core has to be *turned on*. Are you starting to find your deep core? Is it *turned on*?

Bear in mind that it can take time to see alignment changes with deep core activation. However, with the addition of other techniques, not just activating the deep core, I have seen changes occur very fast. Everyone heals in their own time. Also, everyone is in a different stage of body discovery. Seeing a professional is always ideal in my mind's eye, as this can expedite your results. However, don't rely on someone else to fix all of your musculoskeletal problems — keeping the body healthy is a lifestyle. Use the knowledge and insight you do have and gather more! You have one body in this life; treat it with respect and listen to it. It is smart and very connected. Keep the connections going: mind, body, spirit! All have forms of intelligence and all need to work together.

EMPHASIZING THE IMPORTANCE OF A NEUTRAL SPINE

Lie back on a therapy ball, chest up. Your back is now in an arched position (no longer neutral) throughout the spine. This arched position will affect the ability of your extremities to move with ease. Try lifting your legs in this position, one leg, then the other. The deep core cannot fire as easily.

Now come out of the extended position by lifting your head up and your pelvis up to form a neutral spine. Try lifting one of your legs up with your whole spine straight/neutrally aligned over the ball. You should notice improved stability and much less mobility at the pelvis and lower back, as well as an improved ability to lift your legs. You might notice that your legs feel lighter. And you should notice improved activation of the transverse abdominis in neutral spine.

CONNECT THE TRANSVERSE ABDOMINIS TO YOUR POSTURE

Look at every type of professional athlete and you will notice that almost all of them have very good posture. Why is posture important? The deep transverse abdominis muscles fires better when they are aligned and that state of alignment indirectly makes it easier for you to move your extremities. Posture affects your breath, your internal organs, AND your performance. Activate your transverse abdominis to maintain good posture when sitting, walking, squatting, exercising, running, swimming, etc.

- Use this muscle when thinking about posture.
- When should you have good posture? All of the time!

MORE ON TRAINING: MAKE IT A HABIT

You tell your child to clean up their room each day, hoping that they will eventually just do it without being asked. The hoped-for response from your child is much like the hoped-for response of your body's muscles. With effective training, the transverse abdominis muscle will eventually be on habitually. Habits take consistency. Furthermore, you have to train sport specific, in that you have to train the transverse abdominis to work for your personal everyday movements.

Not only does the transverse abdominis muscle need to be strong enough, it also needs to be programmed properly so the brain and body function together smoothly and efficiently. The muscle will take the route it knows — the path that is familiar. So, although the muscle may be strong, if you only train it to turn on while doing squats, it won't necessarily turn on when doing side steps or running. It potentially has a completely different and well-compensated route for this. You must "brain map." *Think about these muscles* with all of your activities to have them WORK FOR YOU.

WALK

Do muscle training all of the time with all of your daily movements. I mean do it a lot! A study published in 2016 supports the idea that walking while doing pelvic floor contractions and abdominal hollowing improves the activation of both the transverse abdominis and the multifidi muscles.[8] I can tell you from personal and clinical experience that this is true.

If the transverse abdominis muscle was turned off or too weak to function with some activities, you will need to thoughtfully create new pathways that activate the transverse abdominis. Again, even if you have trained these muscles and they start to work for you, there will be times when they will want to stop and revert back to old pathways (the ones you had been using to compensate for a weak or dysfunctional transverse abdominis). The more you incorporate the transverse abdominis muscles into your life, with everything you do, the less likely your body is to fall back upon the old mechanics. The brain needs repetition to learn. Mass practice is required with all of the deep core muscles, as noted in both this chapter and the previous chapter.

Again, many times after my patients have identified the pelvic floor and transverse abdominis muscles, I will ask them to activate them with their activities of daily living. For example, I will have them do a squat with their transverse abdominis and pelvic floor muscles contracted. Often, they will say that it is so much easier. The core, when *turned on*, can truly make functional mobility less effort-ful. And, in sport and in life, ease of movement is important.

TRANSVERSE ABDOMINIS AND DIASTASIS RECTI ABDOMINIS

I have found that many females with diastasis recti abdominis focus on exercises aimed at the obliques and rectus abdominis. Sometimes this works and they *do* actually eliminate their diastasis recti abdominis. However, this doesn't work for all females. I believe it depends on the severity of their diastasis recti abdominis and their ability to get tension at the linea alba. Furthermore, it will depend on the mobility of the muscle and fascia at their abdomen, along with the strength and neuromuscular control of their transverse abdominis. Success will also depend on lifestyle; are they getting enough rest, enough healthy food, and enough support to heal after pregnancy? If their transverse abdominis is *turned on* to some degree, or if it turns on with exercises focusing on the obliques and rectus abdominis, then I would expect the tension at the linea alba to develop. Furthermore, I would expect the diastasis recti abdominis and appearance of the abdominals to be improved.

ACTIVATE THE TRANSVERSE ABDOMINIS BY
RELEASING THE MULTIFIDI

Interestingly, when I release tight deep muscles of the back, the transverse abdominis is noted on imaging and with palpation to improve its contractile ability and increased tension is noted at the linea alba. Think about pregnancy: both the linea alba and transverse abdominis thin and elongate to accommodate the baby, and the back commonly goes into increased lordosis (increased arch of the spine into extension). In order to do this, the muscles of the lower back shorten and tighten and, many times, develop trigger points. These trigger points can increase the lordosis and that position alone can pull on the muscles and fascia of the stomach. This could create a diastasis recti abdominis. By releasing the trigger points of the multifidi, you are allowing for less pulling at the front of the body at the skin, muscle, and fascia. Also, by releasing the multifidi you are potentially improving neuronal flow (electrical input from body and the brain) to the muscle as you are increasing the joint spaces. In fact, I find tension at the front and back of the body to be very specific; if the transverse abdominis is weak, for example, at L2 (the second lumbar vertebra), I commonly find a correlating tightness at that level in the back at the multifidi (another deep core muscle we will discuss in the next chapter).

Remember, many variables can affect healing: emotions, lifestyle, rest, the support of family and friends, finances, stress, belief systems. Also, remember that there are good people out there who want to be a part of your team and help you meet your goals! Call on them!

ADDRESS YOUR INTERNAL FORCES

I use the term "internal forces" to refer to forces inside and around your own tissues (bone, fascia, connective tissue, muscle, skin) and the stresses they place on your body. Resting internal forces can be in the form of tension, compression, shear, friction, chemical, physiological, or electrical forces. At rest, your body can be fighting itself. For example, your fascia or muscle could be stuck in a shortened and adhesive manner, therefore restricting your ability to get into a neutral spine position for good posture. As another example, your transverse abdominis might not want to fire if it is bound to your abdominal muscles with scar tissue.

Misalignment in your tissue can amplify forces on your body. For example, tight ligaments, tight retinaculum, and/or a tight capsule of the knee can compress a joint that is not even weight bearing. Think of it like a vice compressing on your joint. This is real. Think of a tight latissimus dorsi muscle — the biggest muscle of the back. It can compress a vast aspect of your spine. Even without the force of gravity, if your latissimus dorsi muscle or its fascia is tight, it can cause compressive forces on your spine and shoulder.

It is important to minimize the number of misalignments and soft tissue imbalances within your body in order to take the load off of the transverse abdominis. Musculoskeletal and fascial imbalances add a layer of personal internal forces that your body has to fight against.

Your internal forces will help to determine how you function statically and dynamically, in general and at your deep core. When adding movement to your internal forces, now they become more dynamic and not static. I like to refer to internal forces at play with movement as dynamic internal forces. An excellent physical therapist or bodyworker can help to align your body's tissues so the deep core can fire more easily and with less internal resistant forces, dynamically and statically.

You don't want to turn on a car and simply proceed to drive it if the drivetrain is not aligned, or the wheels are not balanced, or there is no oil in the engine. All of these oversights would make your car's job much more difficult. You need a mechanic to help you diagnose your car, just as you probably need a physical therapist or a bodyworker for your body.

REFERENCES

1. Cirocchi R, Cheruiyot I, Henry BM, et al. Anatomical variations of the pyramidalis muscle: a systematic review and meta-analysis. *Surgical and Radiologic Anatomy.* 2021;43:595-605.

2. Häggmark T, Thorstensson A. Fibre types in human abdominal muscles. *Acta Physiologica Scandinavica.* 1979;107:319-25. doi:10.1111/j.1748- 1716.1979.tb06482.x

3. Netter FH. *Atlas of Human Anatomy.* 7th ed. Elsevier; 2018.

4. Hernia. Cleveland Clinic. February 7, 2023. Accessed January 3, 2025. https://my.clevelandclinic.org/health/diseases/15757-hernia

5. Rath AM, Attali P, Dumas JL, Goldlust D, Zhang J, Chevrel JP. The abdominal linea alba: an anatomo-radiologic and biomechanical study. *Surgical and Radiologic Anatomy.* 1996;18:281-88. doi:10.1007/BF01627606

6. Boissonnault JS, Blaschak MJ. Incidence of diastasis recti abdominis during the childbearing year. *Physical Therapy.* 1988;68:1082-6. doi:10.1093/ptj/68.7.1082

7. Parker MA, Millar LA, Dugan SA. Diastasis rectus abdominis and lumbo-pelvic pain and dysfunction-are they related? *Journal of Women's Health Physical Therapy.* 2009;33:15-22.

8. Lee AY, Baek SO, Cho YW, Lim TH, Jones R, Ahn SH. Pelvic floor muscle contraction and abdominal hollowing during walking can selectively activate local trunk stabilizing muscles. *Journal of Back and Musculoskeletal Rehabilitation.* 2016;29:731-9. doi:10.3233/BMR-160678

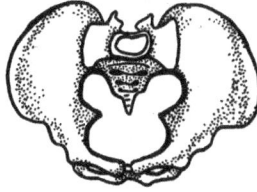

MULTIFIDI

The multifidi muscles are deep in your back, running the entire length of your spine from your sacrum all the way up to the top of your neck to your skull, the occiput. WOW! What other deep muscles do that?

The multifidi are part of the transversospinales muscle group.[1] This group consists of the semispinalis, multifidi, and rotatores. All of these muscles share the same functional movements. The semispinalis muscles are located in the cervical and thoracic vertebrae only. The rotatores *do* span the entire length of the vertebral spine. The inter-transversarii muscles are another group of deep muscles that run between transverse processes of the spine mainly at the cervical and lumbar regions.

The multifidi have been studied more than these other muscles and are more easily identified. They will be the deep spine muscles focused on in this book. My clinical training and studies have been focused on the multifidi. We can identify the multifidi muscles kinesthetically, with palpation, or with real time imaging.

The latissimus dorsi and the erector spinae muscles are superficial to the multifidi. The multifidi attach serially to vertebrae, originating at the transverse processes of your vertebrae and inserting at the spinous processes of your vertebrae two to four vertebral levels above their origin. The multifidi are short fibers with relatively long width. I like to think of these muscles as the perfect bridges connecting the vertebrae — a structurally solid bridge to hold the vertebrae together.

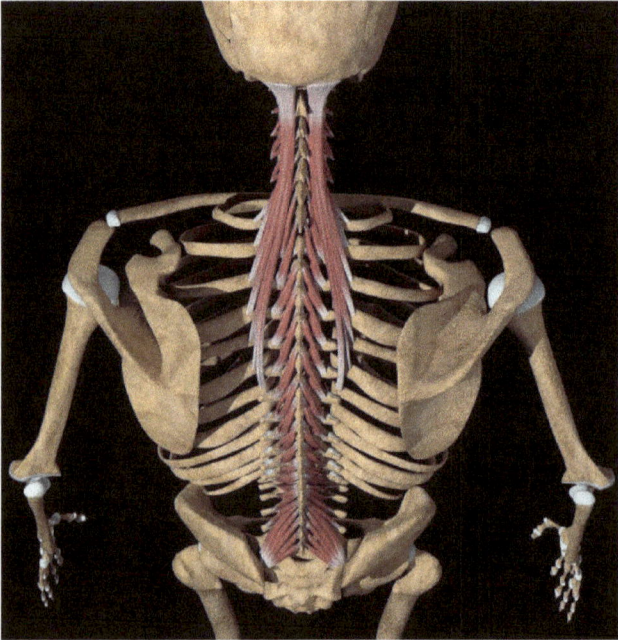

Figure 4.1. Multifidi.
From MadiGraphic/*Shutterstock.com.*

The multifidi create triangular shapes like those found in a truss bridge. Triangles are strong because force is evenly distributed from the vertex to the base of each side of the triangle. A square has a weak spot at the center and collapses more easily. You can see triangles deep within the multifidi (Figure 4.1). The body's structural engineering is amazing! These muscles are small, but very powerful! Let's take a closer look:

Origin: Posterior sacrum (next to foramina), posterior superior iliac spine, mammillary processes of lumbar vertebrae, transverse processes of thoracic vertebrae, articular processes of C4-C7.[1]

Location/Insertion: Spinous processes of vertebrae (except C1/atlas), two to four bones above origin.[1]

Function/Bilateral Action: When the multifidi on both sides of the spine contract, they are assisting with back bending of the spine.

Function/Unilateral Action: When multifidi are working on only one side of the spine, they allow side bending to same side and rotation to opposite side.[2]

Interestingly, the multifidi attach to quite a large portion of your sacrum. Again, the pelvis is often overlooked and the sacral multifidi are not discussed. Considering the mass amount of insertion points for the multifidi onto the sacrum, one could see how restoring range of motion at the sacral multifidi could affect sacral, sacroiliac, and lumbopelvic mobility. In Figure 4.2, the red is outlining the left side of the sacrum where the multifidus is attached. The bulk of the multifidi are at the lumbar sacral region, where stability is crucial. Overall, the multifidi muscular attachments are actually quite expansive.

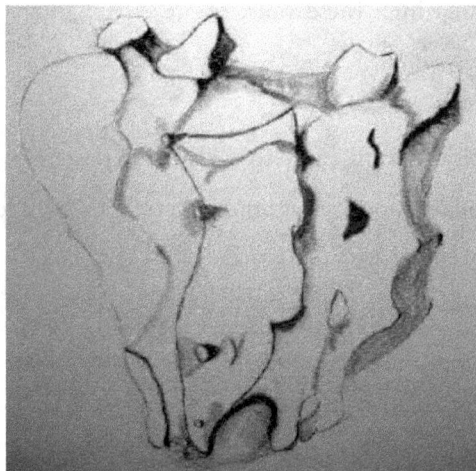

Figure 4.2. Multifidus attachment at the sacrum.
By Renee Zupancich.

WHY SHOULD I STRENGTHEN THE MULTIFIDI?

The multifidi have multiple important functions. The multifidi stabilize the vertebrae, allow segmental mobility of the spine, assist with isolated mobility of the spine, protect the central nervous system, and help preserve the disc space and vertebral joints.

Stable Platform for the Extremities

When the multifidi are aligned and robust, they are able to provide a stable and balanced platform for the extremities and the long muscles of the spine. Remember the multifidi origin and insertion; the small and relatively thick muscles go along the spine in one to four levels at a time. When these muscles are *turned on*, they can stabilize the spine for more dynamic movements of the extremities and/or spine.

Activation of the multifidi supports the extremities by providing a stable base to push off from. Similarly to the other deep core muscles that we have discussed (pelvic floor and transverse abdominis), the multifidi muscles fire ahead of time before any extremity movement occurs. They "act" before the extremities move, preemptively *turning on* to assist with stability for optimal strength.

Imagine a gymnast hanging horizontally from a pole (doing a "human flag"). What if the pole was moving and not a solid and stable object? Think of your spine as the pole and the gymnast as an extremity. If the gymnast tried to hang horizontally from the pole and the pole moved like a rope, it would be much more difficult. They would have no stable surface on which to apply their force. Similarly, if your core is weak, it will make the job of your extremities much more difficult. Not having a functionally strong and mobile deep core will limit your full potential in quality and efficiency of movement and strength.

Spinal Mobility

The spine is known as the vertebral column. There are twenty-six bones in the adult spine: seven cervical bones, twelve thoracic bones, five lumbar bones, the sacrum, and the coccyx. The multifidi act not only to stabilize the joints of the spine, but also to move them. These joints allow for forward bending, backward bending, and twisting.

The spine is like a snake; it allows for a lot of dynamic movement at multiple segments. Furthermore, there is a lot of room for compensation. If one segment or joint becomes immobile, the spine can adapt. However, what happens when multiple adaptations have occurred and when one has run out of compensations at the spine? When this happens, one will have decreased spinal mobility, which may lead to pain as well as poor imaging, not just on X-ray! One might appear bent over, shifted, bent to the side, etc.

Impairments of the back often involve the multifidi atrophying and/or turning off. When moving from sitting to standing, the spine might take multiple seconds or minutes to adjust, and might not even come into alignment. Just like a snake, if the spine locks up mid-way, its slithering mobility will not be so elegant. To me, mobility of the spine is a sign of youth and health. It is an attractive body part, often dictating the health of the whole body! One of the first ways someone will describe the physical appearance of an elderly person is "all bent over." So, if one wants to rejuvenate themselves, take a look at the spine and the multifidi.

Protection of the Central Nervous System

The multifidi also protect the central nervous system, keeping your brain connected to your spinal cord. Without the central nervous system staying connected, we can become paralyzed.

The brain and spinal cord make up the central nervous system. I believe the body is involved in a constant state of effort to keep the spinal cord connected to the brain and to keep the spinal cord connected to itself. The multifidi are some of the closest and deepest muscles to assist in this process.

The body responds to trauma in a protective fashion. For example, patients who have had whiplash from a motor vehicle accident will often have significantly tight cervical and upper thoracic musculature and fascia. The multifidi are often affected and can present as tight. With time, the multifidi can even present as deactivated and/or atrophied. If you think about it, the body has done its job. The body kept the central nervous system together through the accident. This is a good thing, however, people often become stuck in a protective position following injury. Individuals may become unable to use their deep muscles functionally and therefore compromise their spinal and/or extremity mobility. The multifidi are then at risk of becoming turned off or stuck in an *on* position. The multifidi are not coiling and recoiling from a lengthened and shortened position anymore. They are often tight and weak. If left untreated long enough, they are at risk of atrophy.

Knowing how to identify and activate the deep core muscles is a very important part of recovery from accidents, but is also important in day-to-day life. Prolonged sitting can be just as bad as, sometimes worse than, being in a motor vehicle accident.

As I have said, fascia and muscle tend to stay in a contracted position following injury or trauma in order to protect a healing area. This is not just the case at the deep core. For example, after injuring my achilles tendon, I decided to release my gastrocnemius and soleus muscle only to have increased tension, pain, and inflammation at the site of injury. *At what time* we release fascia and activate muscle matters for healing. Everyone heals in their own time; we are all unique and in different situations that will affect our healing.

Knowing your deep core, when it is working and not working for you, can help you in your healing journey. Check your systems! Is your deep core system intact? Simple imagery following an accident or injury does not show this. You will need a qualified physical therapist or real time imaging to assess your deep core. This book can also help you assess your deep core!

Factors that may adversely affect healing include: financial restraints, family situations, lack of time or willingness to rest, economic stress, inability to take time off from work, lack of ability to obtain skilled bodywork, lack of quality clinicians, improper medication, poor diet, stress, mental inability to "let go", etc. Another thing that adversely affects healing is lack of knowledge, especially knowledge about your body, specifically the deep core!

We all require something a little different at different times in our healing. I cannot tell you how many times patients have been told by doctors, "You are just going to have to live with it; it has been months and/or years and that is how it is going to be." This is just all too often not true. The body is adaptable and capable of healing with the right treatments, rest, modalities, support, *knowledge*, etc.

Decompression of the Spine

The multifidi muscles assist in providing a supported space between the vertebrae of the spine. The spinal nerves emerge from the spinal column through an opening between adjacent vertebrae. This space is important as it allows nerves to travel out of the spinal cord to the body for axonal flow — electrical and chemical flow that allows sensory input from the body to the brain and motor output from the brain to the body. When the multifidi are healthy and have full mobility and strength, they are like mini shock absorbers assisting in prevention of compression of the vertebral joints.

When an individual is weak in their deep multifidi muscles, they will feel the vertebral joint spaces being compressed. These individuals will often describe this feeling as a sharp pain. The pain often occurs during momentary compression, usually with unexpected movements and forces on vertebral joint spaces. If compression is happening continuously, in part due to weak multifidi, there can be motor and sensory nerve impingements. Sometimes the multifidi are weak and the nerves are not notably affected; these individuals can present with achy back pain. Achy back pain is clinically seen as consistent forces and inflammation at the vertebral joint spaces. Restoring the multifidi often restores segmental mobility and strength, decreasing the inflammation.

When the multifidi muscles are in a shortened position, they are technically shortening the distance between your vertebrae. That shortened position can act like a vise, compressing the joint spaces. With a shortened distance between the vertebrae, one is at risk of pinching off or entrapping the spinal nerves. When the length of the multifidi is restored, then the spine becomes decompressed.

Activation of the multifidi can assist in treating and preventing common diagnoses at the intervertebral joints of the spine. Degenerative disc disease (DDD), stenosis, herniated discs, bulged discs, protruded discs, and osteoarthritis of the cartilage at intervertebral joint surfaces are some examples. These diagnoses can make someone feel really old and *not* mobile. Support the spine with your multifidi — that's what they are for! Is your spine being supported? Are your multifidi muscles *turned on?*

HYPERMOBILITY AND HYPOMOBILITY

With instability at the spine, the intervertebral joints are often either hypermobile (moving too much) or hypomobile (moving too little). Sometimes the unstable joints become compressed from the tight and therefore limited functional mobility of the multifidi, thus creating hypomobility and lack of axonal flow and blood flow. Other times the multifidi are atrophied, causing hypermobility and a shift or bend in the spine secondary to lack of strength of the multifidi muscles.

Mobility is not always a sign that the multifidi are *on;* the spine can hinge in segments, making it appear that you have normal mobility to the untrained eye. A hypermobile segment of the spine often has underdeveloped multifidi muscles and an abnormal amount of movement. Without the support of *turned on* multifidi muscles, one is risking excessive forces at that joint and/or surrounding joints.

The multifidi may also be overworked at the segments of the spine above and/or below a weak spot. Hypertrophy, or overdevelopment of the muscles, can happen. Often these spots appear hypermobile. The weak link of the spine is not at the hypermobile spot; rather, the hypermobile spot is compensating for a weak link at a higher or lower segment of the spine. There is an overdevelopment occurring to compensate for the weakness above or below it. Clinically, this can present as a horizontal band of hypertrophic muscle, commonly seen in the lower lumbar. A classical weak lower core leads to overdevelopment of the mid back along with pain at the mid back and/or lower and upper back.

Just like with other weak core muscles, it is common for the muscles of the extremities to compensate for weak multifidi. For example, the hip flexors and/or the hip rotator muscles can become overworked. The long muscles of the spine are another common compensation for weak multifidi. The body may also create stability with fascia. Fascia can contract. There are many ways the body may choose to compensate, and compensations are not always consistent; the body can change its compensatory strategies. Clinically, patients will say their pain has moved or moves, and this inconsistency can make patients feel hypocritical and question their pain altogether.

DRY NEEDLING THE MULTIFIDI

Dry needling the multifidi is one way to restore function and mobility. Dr. Gunn is one of the pioneers of dry needling and has coined the term intramuscular stimulation. He believes that "myofascial pain syndrome is always a result of peripheral neuropathy or radiculopathy."[3] He defines myofascial pain syndrome as "a condition that causes disordered function in the peripheral nerve," based on Cannon and Rosenblueth's "Law of Denervation," which states that the function and integrity of innervation structures is dependent upon the free flow of nerve impulses to provide a regulatory or trophic effect.[3,4] Dr. Gunn is known for heavily dry needling the multifidi to open peripheral nerve pathways along the spine. The theory is that tight and shortened multifidi are potentially the cause of peripheral neuropathy and radiculopathy and denervation. Clinically I have found this to be true. And honestly this makes logical and simple sense. I do love the immediate and sometimes profoundly good effects that dry needling can have, especially at the multifidi. However, I do not believe that myofascial pain is always a result of peripheral neuropathy.

HOW DO YOU KNOW IF THE MULTIFIDI ARE TURNED ON?

No Back Pain from Occiput to Sacrum

One good sign that you are *turned on* is if you have no back pain. You do not have stiffness at the end of the day or random jabs of pain with small or big movements, specifically unexpected movements. You are able to lie down on your back and stomach without pain or stiffness. Pain is definitely not in and of itself a means to determine if you are *turned on,* however. In fact, numerous patients with significantly dysfunctional backs have no pain, yet the multifidi are nonexistent (completely atrophied) or severely weak.

Good Mobility in the Spine

Good spinal mobility is a sign that the multifidi are *turned on*. Is each segment of your spine moving? Are you able to control the segmental movement of each vertebra? Specifically, can you stand with your knees slightly bent and move your vertebrae segmentally from your head to your sacrum? Try this by standing and bending one vertebra at a time, starting from your neck and ending at your sacrum. Assess where your mobility is coming from by attempting to feel segmental mobility at each vertebra at a time. Do you have the ability to feel each vertebra move? Another sign of good mobility is segmental movement of the spine into flexion (bending) and extension (straightening) when performing sit-ups. Good rotation is another sign. Can you sit with your sit bones planted and segmentally rotate to each side equally and with full range?

Muscle Bulk

You can palpate the multifidi to identify some bulk of the muscle. Generally speaking, if the multifidi muscles have some bulk, they are being used and are *turned on*. However, they may be overused or un coordinated. Furthermore, if the muscles were recently turned off, they may have some bulk, as the atrophy is not obvious. Palpation is discussed further in a later section of this chapter.

Good Alignment of the Spine

The multifidi help to align the spine. When the multifidi are *turned on,* the spine is often aligned. And when the spine is aligned, there is often symmetry of the deep core muscles.

If the multifidi are asymmetrical, then the spine is often seen as misaligned to some degree. This is often the case in patients with scoliosis and in patients presenting with a curved spine or a shift in the spine. This is also commonly the case in patients with excessive kyphosis (forward bending of the spine) and/or lordosis (backward bending of the spine). If the asymmetry in the multifidi is multi-segmental, in that there are multiple levels of vertebrae where the multifidi are turned off, weak, or immobile, then misalignment of the spine is more likely.

Good Transverse Abdominis Strength

If the transverse abdominis is weak, the multifidi are often also weak at the same level within the spine. The transverse abdominis is often activated to assist in the firing of the multifidi, which is not surprising as these muscles are connected via fascia. It can also be helpful to release the multifidi to assist in the firing of the transverse abdominis at the same level.

No Overly Tight Fascia Along the Long Muscles of the Back

Often the long muscles of the spine appear to compensate for weak deep and superficial multifidi. It is common to see overly active and developed long muscles and fascia of the spine with weak multifidi lying underneath. These muscles and fascia may be painful and spasm when the deep core is weak. Remember, the long muscles of the spine and the latissimus dorsi can act to compress the spine and can potentially disrupt the function and strength of the multifidi. They can take over the job of the multifidi and/or make it hard for the multifidi to activate. Loosening the long muscles and fascia of the spine can assist with multifidi, and all deep core muscle, activation.

No Swelling Along the Spine

An absence of swelling along the spine is a sign that the multifidi are *turned on*. Remember, the multifidi act as little shock absorbers for the spine and also assist with alignment. They fire before movement occurs in order to stabilize and protect the spine. If there is swelling, it is a sign that unnecessary forces are being applied to the spine and the vertebral joints are being compressed.

HOW DO YOU KNOW IF THE MULTIFIDI ARE *TURNED OFF?*

Pain

Pain might be a sign that the multifidi are turned off or are weak. Numerous other ailments and issues can cause low back pain. However, generally, the main cause of recurring low back pain is weakness of the back muscles.[5] Clinically, this is very common.

Decreased Muscle Bulk

Decreased bulk or atrophy of the multifidi can be another sign that the muscles are not firing or are weak or dysfunctional. Ultrasound can be useful to observe the cross-sectional area of the back muscles at the lower lumbar and the sacrum. Asymmetry of the multifidi muscles is frequently found at the lumbar spine. This is also a common site for low back pain and spinal injury.

Lack of Movement in the Spine

Lack of movement in the spine is another sign the multifidi might be turned off. If no movement is occurring at a particular segment of the spine, it could be the case that shortened, locked up, or "off" multifidi are restricting the range of motion.

Radicular Symptoms

Radicular symptoms include numbness, tingling, itching, or burning. Radiculopathy may be caused by compression, inflammation, and/or injury to the spinal nerve. Disc lesions are a common cause of lumbosacral radiculopathy and may be related to multifidi atrophy. Which came first? The disc lesion or the weak multifidi? In patients with one-sided lumbosacral radiculopathy, Hyun et al. reported a significant decrease in the cross-sectional area of the multifidus muscle located on the same side as the radiculopathy.[6]

Tight multifidi or other back muscles may cause compression

of a nerve or joint space. Again, what came first — the nerve being damaged and the muscle turning off, or the muscle turning off or tightening, causing nerve damage? Was there a misalignment that caused the muscle to turn off, or did misalignment follow the muscle turning off? Either way, identifying and activating the multifidi will be a great start to healing and improved alignment.

No Obvious Sign

There may be no obvious sign that the multifidi are turned off. You may feel and see nothing. However, for the trained eye, there are usually clues if the multifidi are turned off or are too tight and limiting a normal state of functioning. One way to discover this is with palpation. Another way to assess the multifidi is with ultrasound-guided therapy.

Swelling

Swelling is an indication that the multifidi are turned off or are not working to their full potential. When swelling occurs, the body is unable to transmit electrical impulses or respond via electrical impulses as effectively. A swollen joint does not respond as quickly due to boggy information. Swelling can then lead to atrophy due to lack of use. But which came first? Did the multifidi turn off, leading to swelling? Or did the swelling happen first?

When compression, shear, or tensile forces place too much physical stress on joints or tissues within the body, swelling and inflammation can occur. Weakness or imbalance in tissues and muscles can lead to direct or indirect forces along the spine. Musculoskeletal and fascial conditions, medical conditions, and emotional, physiological, and spiritual imbalances can also impact the forces on the spine.

If the multifidi are turned off or are too tight, this can lead to excessive forces at the spine. When the multifidi are not able to adequately support the vertebral joints, multiple forces are allowed to come between the joints. These forces can cause increased stress on the joints and tissue at individual or at multiple segments of the spine. These forces can then lead to inflammation in the tissue and in the bone.

Excessive forces can also *cause* the multifidi muscles to turn off. For example, if you fall onto your tailbone or if you deadlift too much weight, the multifidi could be injured. Repetitive low load can also cause fatigue and failure of the deep and superficial multifidi, leading to inflammation. Repetitive motion seen with labor workers and athletes can cause low load fatigue and eventually failure of the multifidi. Swelling is often seen in conjunction with the failure of the multifidi.

One could speculate that swelling, atrophy of the multifidi, and inflammation could cause pain, disc lesions, radiculopathy, spinal stenosis, scoliosis, or poor musculoskeletal alignment. Swelling slows the conduction of electrical impulses, and as a result, the multifidi may no longer activate, leading to a shift or bend in the back.

USE THE MULTIFIDI TO DECREASE SWELLING

Movement and activation of the multifidi muscles can help to de-crease swelling. Movement brings improved blood flow and nutrients to the affected tissue. This is the reason why I tell people to walk twenty to forty-five minutes a day, to increase blood flow to the mus-cles and joints and to decrease day-to-day swelling caused by com-pression of the spine. Walking allows the long muscles of the spine to relax and lengthen from a long day of work or play.

Sometimes walking is too much load for one's back. In that case, try swimming with fins or crawling (remember to protect your knees). If this is too much, rest and seek the aid of a qualified profes-sional. Bodywork is almost always helpful at all stages of healing, provided you have a good bodyworker!

The following sections will assist you in identifying your multifidi muscles and *turning them on*. Remember, activating the multifidi can assist with reducing inflammation and improving alignment.

HOW CAN YOU PALPATE THESE MUSCLES THAT ARE SO DEEP?

There are a few ways that you can palpate the multifidi muscles. These muscles run the length of your spine from the cranium to the sacrum. A good place to palpate these muscles is in your lower back, in the lumbar region. Start by finding your spinous processes (the bony prominences that run along the center of your spine) and palpate (feel) immediately to the left and right (Figure 4.3). Keep your fingers at this location for the following assessments.

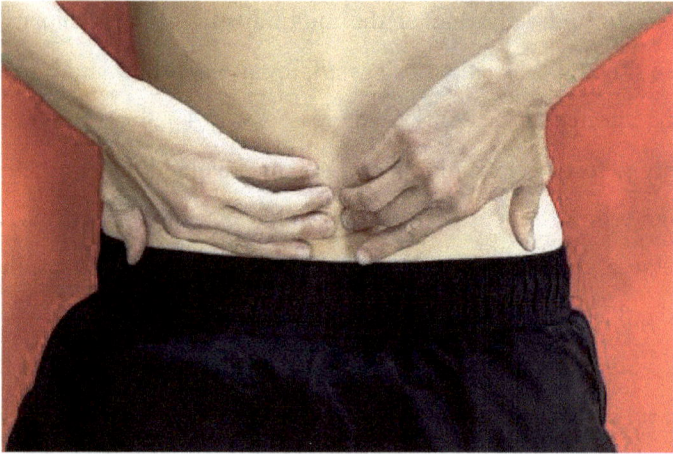

Figure 4.3. Palpate immediately to the left and right of the spinous processes.

You can assess the multifidi in any position; below are just a few examples. When you are assessing, try to compare the left and right sides. Start at your sacrum and work your way up to your mid thoracic multifidi as far as you can reach. Mid thoracic can be hard to reach for most people. Then start again from the occiput (the back of the skull) to feel the cervical multifidi (in the neck) and move your fingers down to the upper thoracic (upper back) to complete the rest of spine as you are able.

Here are some things to feel for:

- The quality of the muscle should be firm, not mushy.
- The muscle should fill the space along either side of the spinous processes (there should not be a hole).
- The muscle should not be painful to touch.
- The muscle should be symmetrical to the left and right.
- The muscle should fire milliseconds prior to any movement of the extremities.

SITTING: Sit up straight. Tighten your transverse abdominis (see chapter "Transverse Abdominis"). Just by sitting up you might feel the lumbar multifidi of the lower back activate. This will feel like a firm swelling into your fingers, like your bicep when you flex it, but at a much smaller level. Next, lift some of the weight off of one of your feet while still keeping the foot on the ground. Again, you should be able to feel an even bigger "swell" of muscle into your fingers. The swell should be bigger on the side opposite of the lifted leg.

WALKING: With good posture, and by lightly tightening your transverse abdominis, you should feel your left lower lumbar multifidi activate prior to your left hip extension and right hip flexion each time that you bring your right leg forward. Each time that you bring your left leg forward, you should feel your right lower lumbar multifidi activate prior to right hip extension and left hip flexion.

LYING DOWN: Lie on your stomach. Again, maintain good posture.

Many people cannot lie on their stomach with good posture. You might want to put a thinner pillow under your abdomen at your waist. This supports tight lumbar/pelvis/hip joints. Now lift your left leg. You should feel the lower lumbar multifidi activate. You should feel a bigger swell on the right, opposite of the leg lifted.

HOW DO YOU *TURN ON* THE MULTIFIDI MUSCLES?

Watch your posture during the following exercises and always try to put yourself in neutral spine. This might require pillows or props to support poor posture that is in a non-neutral position. This might also require a chin tuck or posterior or anterior pelvic tilt to open up the vertebral spaces. Try to take the stress off of the multifidi by opening up the space where the multifidi are trying to activate. Make sure that any muscles that might be pulling the spine out of alignment are relaxed and in a position that will not make them activate or further pull on the spine. Place your hands on either side of the spinous processes to assure activation of the multifidi with the below exercises.

MULTIFIDI ACTIVATION AT ALL LEVELS OF THE SPINE: NECK, UPPER BACK, LOWER BACK, AND SACRUM

Place one finger above the level of multifidi you are trying to activate and another finger below. Now think of tensioning that space between your two fingers. This usually involves lengthening your spine between the targeted vertebrae. Imagine a bow and arrow — drawing the space between your two fingers like the string on a bow. Contract the multifidi and the muscle should swell into the space. You can think about making a "taut band" between the vertebrae with the multifidi.

CERVICAL SPINE MULTIFIDI ACTIVATION

While Sitting

Imagine your neck long, with space between your cervical vertebrae. Rotate your head to the left and nod up and down. Try not to nod more than five millimeters up and down for five to ten repetitions. Then attempt to move only one millimeter up and down. Precision often requires increased muscle recruitment from the deep core multifidi and the deep core cervical flexors, which assist to open the vertebral spaces. Repeat to the other side.

While Lying Down

Lie on your back with your back flat. Prepare to lift up the weight of your head, as if you *were going* to lift your head off of the floor. This initiation should engage the deep cervical muscles along either side of the throat in the front of the neck, which will assist in opening the cervical vertebrae. Then rotate your head slightly to the right (less than twenty degrees) and attempt to nod a few millimeters up and down. This should assist to activate the cervical multifidi. Repeat to the other side.

LUMBAR SPINE MULTIFIDI ACTIVATION

Using the Transverse Abdominis

One way to turn on the multifidi is to use the transverse abdominis. Simply activate the transverse abdominis and feel for the multifidi. Again, maintaining good posture is key to assist in activating the deep core. Try sitting, lying prone (on the stomach), side-lying, or quadruped (on hands and knees). Focus on activating the transverse abdominis at the same vertebral level as the section of multifidi you are trying to activate. Imagine the vertebral segments separating in a bowing manner.

Side-Lying Palpation With Perturbation

You can activate your transverse abdominis muscle and then repetitively push or tap on the multifidi you are attempting to activate. Try to make the taps short and fast. It is important to activate the transverse abdominis at the same level you are trying to activate the multifidi. Start with two- to ten-second contractions of the multifidi. Attempt six sets of ten a day for mass practice. An ideal position to start in is side-lying with knees bent to ninety degrees.

Lifting the Upper Extremities in Hook-Lying Position

Lie on your back with your knees bent. Activate your lower abdominals and transverse abdominis. Focusing on the vertebral segments at which you are attempting to activate the multifidi. Then lift your arm (shoulder flexion) as far as you can without leaving neutral spine position. Common compensations for shoulder flexion are flaring of the ribs or arching of the back. Feel for the multifidi to fire milliseconds prior to the arm being lifted. You can also do this in quadruped position (on hands and knees).

Lifting the Lower Leg in Hook-Lying Position

Lie flat on your back with your knees bent. Activate your lower abdominals and then lift one of your lower legs while keeping the knee in a bent position. Progression in this position would be lengthening the leg (which adds weight to the deep core). You can progress as you are able, as long as you are able to keep your transverse abdominis and multifidi *turned on* and you can maintain a neutral spine.

Quadruped

On your hands and knees, slide one leg back to full knee extension while keeping your other knee on the floor. Make sure your sliding foot can smoothly glide; any resistance will make the task more difficult. If the multifidi are weak and just getting *turned on* again, it is important to start with the weight they can handle. Progression in this position would be lifting the foot and moving the leg back to full knee extension while keeping the targeted multifidi activated.

Remember, activate the transverse abdominis to assist in *turning on* the multifidi. Imagine a taut band between the vertebrae of the multifidi you are trying to activate. Maintain good posture to assist in activating the multifidi.

Transverse Abdominis Activation with Opposite Arm Resistance

Stand with good posture in front of a wall. Then activate your transverse abdominis forcefully and push on the wall with the hand opposite of the multifidi you are trying to activate. Remember to keep good posture.

Transverse Abdominis Activation with Arm Resistance
and Perturbation

Stand in the same position as above, activate your transverse abdominis, and push into the wall with the hand opposite of the multifidi you are trying to activate. With the other hand, use one finger to quickly tap on the multifidi you are trying to activate. This is my favorite; it combines three activation exercises into one!

Keep the multifidi activated while progressing through the following more advanced exercises:

- On all fours, really move the leg in any direction while keeping the multifidi activated.
- Add weights, bands, or resistance to the above exercises.
- Add an unstable surface to the above exercises.
- Crawl on hands and knees or bear crawl. Crawling makes it easier for the multifidi to fire, as the load of the body is not segmentally stacked at the vertebral bodies. Make sure the surface you are crawling on is soft and your knees are protected; lush grass or carpet is ideal, along with knee pads.

SEEK PHYSICAL THERAPY WITH A PROFESSIONAL EXPERIENCED IN DEEP CORE ACTIVATION

- Dry needling with electrical stimulation is probably the easiest way to both release and activate the multifidi, if seeing a therapist qualified in these skills.
- Ultrasound-guided activation of the multifidi is another technique that really helps the patient see and understand, and therefore recruit the multifidi more easily.
- Hands-on manual therapy techniques can also be used by experienced practitioners.
- Practitioners with experience with the deep core muscles can help position you for success.

- It is easier to identify the multifidi while holding your breath. As with all deep core activation exercises, you can take out your breath to assist in identifying and initiating the coordination of the multifidi muscles. When you take the breath out, it quiets movement throughout the body and you can better feel the muscle attempting to activate. Obviously, you need to breathe and incorporate the breath back into the exercises later.

- Gravity (standing, sitting) is harder than anti-gravity (lying on the back, stomach, or sides). Gravity can act as a weight and tends to add to poor body mechanics, making activation of the deep core more difficult.

- Sitting is normally more challenging than lying down.

- Standing is more progressive than sitting.

- Adding weight to your body is more progressive than no weight.

- Dynamic positions are considered more progressive than stable positions.

- Walking is more dynamic than standing.

- Running is more dynamic than walking.

REMEMBER: Misalignment and posture also impact the ability of the multifidi to fire. One cannot simply trust that this general list of progressions will work for every person. There are cases where individuals can fire the deep core in the most progressive position listed, but not while lying down.

CARDIO EXERCISES FOR THE MULTIFIDI

Walking and swimming are my "go to" cardio exercises for endurance training of the multifidi muscles. Crawling is also great. If your multifidi or lower core is weak, start swimming with a nice pair of swim fins to maximize the use of the deep core. Also, constantly make sure the multifidi are firing. If the muscles fatigue, take a rest — lie down or use the above exercises to re-activate the multifidi. Keep them on! Constantly remind them that they need to work for you all the time like they are supposed to!

GLOBAL TRAINING EXERCISES TO PROGRESS THE MULTIFIDI ONCE THEY ARE *TURNED ON*

Make sure the multifidi are *turned on* during the below exercises. You can use form as a tool for progression. If you cannot keep your form, modify the exercises (less resistance, less time, etc.).

Lumbar and Thoracic Multifidi Exercises

- Dead Lifts: Start with no weight and good form.
- Bridges: Start with double leg bridges and progress to single leg.
- Squats: Start with no weight and good form.
- Prone hip extension: On your stomach, lift your leg up.
- Prone thoracic extension: On your stomach, bring your chest up.
- Pilates exercises on a mat and reformer: On a reformer, changing the platform, springs, and straps can challenge the deep multifidi.

Pilates in general is probably the best "type" of exercise for the deep core when done with good form. Pilates can help to turn the deep core on, however, not always! You need to KNOW if you are *turned on* first! I've seen some interesting compensations in some very avid pilates students and instructors.

Thoracic and Cervical Multifidi Exercises

- Sitting cervical rotation with one centimeter head nods: While sitting, rotate the head. Start at twenty to thirty degrees of rotation and progress to forty degrees. Nod your head one centimeter up and down ten times in a row. Repeat six times a day. Tap the multifidi along the cervical spine to make sure they are *turned on.*
- Chin tucks in supine: Lie on your back and complete ten chin tucks. Hold each chin tuck for one to three seconds. Repeat six times a day. Progress to ten twenty-second chin tucks, six times a day.
- Chin tucks in prone: Lie on your stomach and complete ten chin tucks. Hold each chin tuck for one to three seconds. Repeat six times a day. Progress to ten twenty-second chin tucks, six times a day.
- Quadruped chin tucks: On all fours, complete ten chin tucks. Hold each chin tuck for one to three seconds. Repeat six times a day. Progress to ten twenty-second chin tucks, six times a day.
- Prone on elbow chin tucks: Lie on your stomach with your elbows beneath your shoulders and your forearms on the ground. Complete ten one- to three-second chin tucks. Repeat six times a day.

day. Progress to ten twenty-second chin tucks, six times a day.

All too often we have health care practitioners, yoga instructors, pilates instructors, and athletic trainers telling their clients, patients, or athletes different positions to put the pelvis in. The most common argument I hear from professionals is that the patient didn't maintain their lumbar lordosis. I believe that *the correct position is closest to where the patient can get both the transverse abdominis and multifidi to turn on.* So, make sure the transverse abdominis and multifidi are both activated while performing exercises. Whether the spine is in neutral, flexion, extension or rotation, these muscles should be firing. It truly is a little different for everyone.

If the deep core is not firing, you are not strengthening the deep core. If you need to go into excessive posterior pelvic tilt to get the deep core to fire, then that is what you need to do. Still, one should ponder why they are unable to fire the deep core in what appears to be a more neutral position. Try to look at the body and its parts relative to each other. Often the problem lies in fascial and muscular restrictions within the body. Sometimes that excessive posterior tilt is actually putting the torso into a more neutral position. When you are aligned at the spine your deep core will fire better!

I observed a class my son took with an Olympian swimmer. The Olympian taught two starting positions — both required a neutral spine, which activated the deep core. With a neutral spine and activated deep core, the swimmers were able to provide a stable plat-

MULTIFIDI   167

form at their pelvis for their legs to push and pull from off the blocks. Posture does matter, and it should be perfected.

HOW DO THE MULTIFIDI RELATE TO ME?

The multifidi muscles are a group of deep core muscles that help us stay aligned, enhance our reaction time, improve our agility and mobility, and provide stability. We want to have good posture and alignment so our body and mind can function. Remember, the multifidi form strong, supportive, dynamic triangles down the spine. The multifidi support the vertebral joint spaces for mobility and stability. These short muscles allow the spine to STABILIZE in multiple segments simultaneously or in isolated segments.

Furthermore, the multifidi allow supported, small segmental MOVEMENT in isolated segments and in multiple segmental and global movements of the spine. The multifidi also act to DECOMPRESS the spine. This decompression also assists in keeping the vertebral joint surfaces from being compressed. When the vertebral joints become compressed, the spine is at risk of degenerative disc disease, osteoarthritis of the vertebral joints, radiculopathy, etc.

Strengthening the multifidi can assist in *prevention and in treatment of spinal diagnoses and symptoms.* We don't want to have pain. Plus, appearance, come on! The spine is sexy, and mobility and flexibility are a TURN ON. A healthy spine is truly a sign of good health. *Really, a healthy spine is the deep core working in harmony!* There is a lot of potential at the spine.

In summary, the multifidi assist with support and stability, agility, mobility, strength, posture, coordination, and alignment. All of these things are needed for sport. When I look at some of the best athletes, their deep core muscles are working with full potential. Of course, they also have other things going for them, including a good training plan, strength and flexibility training, good genes, discipline, mental aptitude, respect for their body, exceptional bodyworkers, coaches, psychologists, financial freedom, good family or support systems, rest, etc., to compete at high levels. But in this book, we are focusing on the deep core as one way to get an edge in life and sport.

The multifidi muscles should naturally be firing with movement. However, it is good to check for optimal performance! Are you *turned on*? That is what this book is about, identifying and attempting to activate the deep core with imagery, cuing, and activation exercises. However, if you cannot or do not understand this book or your body, please seek professional guidance.

REFERENCES

1. Gray H. *Anatomy of the Human Body*. 20th ed. Lea and Febiger; 1918. Accessed April 28, 2025. https://archive.org/details/anatomyofhumanbo1918gray/mode/2up

2. Drake RL, Vogl AW, Mitchell AWM. *Gray's Anatomy for Students*. 2nd ed. London: Churchill Livingstone; 2009.

3. Kalichman L, Vulfsons S. Dry needling in the management of musculoskeletal pain. *Journal of the American Board of Family*

Medicine. 2010;23:640-646. doi:10.3122/
jabfm.2010.05.090296

4. Gunn CC. Radiculopathic pain: Diagnosis and treatment of
    segmental irritation or sensitization. *Journal of Musculoskeletal
    Pain.* 1997;5:119-34. doi:10.1300/J094v05n04_11

5. Lee HJ, Lim WH, Park J, et al. The relationship between cross
    sectional area and strength of back muscles in patients with
    chronic low back pain. *Annals of Rehabilitation Medicine.*
    2012;36:173-181. doi:10.5535/arm.2012.36.2.173

6. Hyun JK, Lee JY, Lee SJ, Jeon JY. Asymmetric atrophy of
    multifidus muscle in patients with unilateral lumbosacral
    radiculopathy. *Spine.* 2007;32:E598-602. doi:10.1097/
    BRS.0b013e318155837b

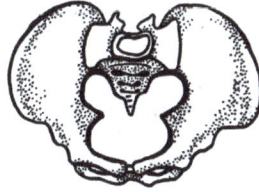

INTERCOSTALS

The intercostal muscles are located between your ribs. Think about the meat on a rack of barbecued ribs (Figure 5.1). When you eat a rack of ribs, you want to have thick, juicy meat between the bones. In your body, you want the intercostal muscles to be strong, with some bulk, and to fill the space between the rib bones. You want the intercostal muscles to be able to coil and recoil to bring rich, oxygenated blood and life to your body. How juicy are your intercostal muscles?

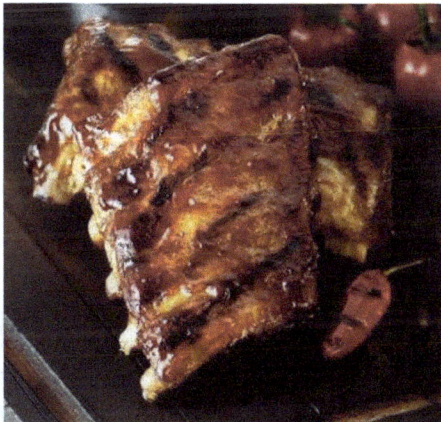

Figure 5.1. The intercostal muscles are the meat between the rib bones.
Adapted from Stockcreations/*Shutterstock.com.*

The human body has twelve ribs. Your ribs start under your clavicle (your collar bone) and go all the way down to a couple of inches above your iliac crest (the top of your pelvis). So the intercostal muscles cover a vast majority of your trunk (see Figure 5.2).

The true ribs, ribs one through seven, begin at the vertebrae of the spine and insert directly onto the sternum via their own cartilage.

Ribs eight through ten are known as false ribs. They attach to the cartilage of rib seven and that cartilage attaches to the sternum. The attachments of ribs eight through ten are therefore not as stable or rigid as the attachments of ribs one through seven.

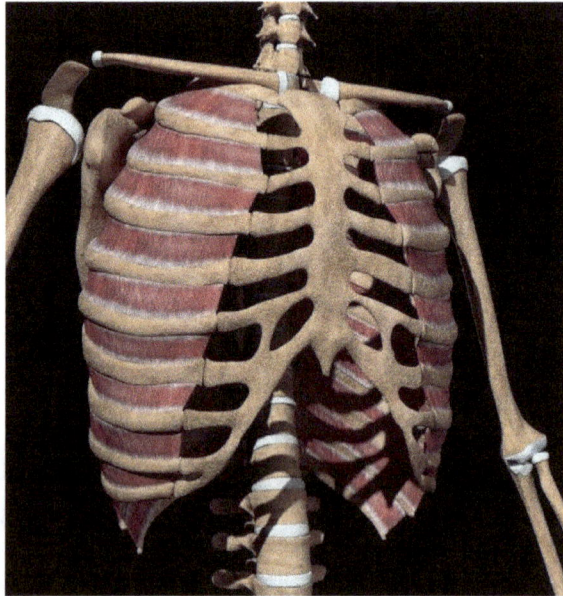

Figure 5.2. The intercostal muscles cover a vast majority of the trunk. From MadiGraphic/*Shutterstock.com.*

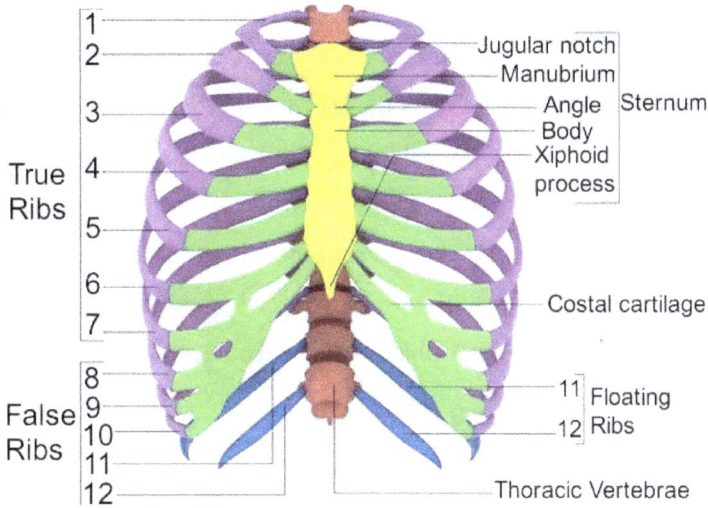

Figure 5.3. Thoracic skeleton anatomy: anterior view.
Adapted from Magic mine/*Shutterstock.com*.

The bottom two ribs, eleven and twelve, are free floating. These two ribs start at the vertebrae at thoracic spine levels eleven and twelve and do not attach to bone or cartilage at the front of the body. Rib eleven commonly ends at your sides. Rib twelve is shorter and a little more on the backside of your body (see Figure 5.3). You can find these floating ribs by putting your hands on your iliac crests and sliding them straight up; you will hit a bone, which is rib eleven. At rib eleven, you can palpate to the end of the bone, which is felt as a nodule that ends, unlike rib ten, which continues to the front side of your body.

Sometimes the ribs can go all the way down *into* the pelvis. This can be seen in people with shortened/tightened/atrophied low back muscles, arthritic vertebrae, and decreased disc spaces. Obviously you do not want your ribs to end up in your pelvis. And yes, I have seen this numerous times. For this reason, remember to think long when doing core exercises and do not to depend on your side muscles (quadratus lumborum and obliques) to compensate for weak and/or tight hips or a weak deep core. Furthermore, don't lock up your abdominals to appear thinner or stronger. This will just compress your joints and bring your ribs closer to the pelvis if done frequently. Stay long! Think long spine! And let your core come to end ranges. Mobilize your core!

UPPER, MIDDLE, AND LOWER
INTERCOSTAL MUSCLES AND RIBS

Therapists who work with the intercostal muscles and ribs often separate them into the upper, middle, and lower intercostal muscles and/ or ribs. We also separate them into front and back and left and right. Start to focus on the quality of your intercostal muscles. As you will learn later, there are specific exercises that can be done to enhance each area.

- Upper intercostal muscles and ribs: T1–T3.
- Middle intercostal muscles and ribs: T4–T7.
- Lower intercostal muscles and ribs: T8–T12.

The majority of *mobility* at the ribs occurs in the lower ribs rather than the upper ribs. In part, this is because the lower ribs are more indirectly connected to the sternum via cartilage or not connected at all. Cartilaginous tissue is designed to allow for some mobility and some stability.

Ribs two through nine each articulate at three locations on each side of your vertebral bodies posteriorly. These connections form two joints on each side of your vertebrae: the costovertebral joints and the costotransverse joints.[1,2] For example, the costovertebral joints of rib seven connect to both the inferior costal facet of vertebra six and the corresponding superior costal facet of rib seven. The costotransverse joints of rib seven are formed via the tubercle on the neck of the rib and the transverse process of the corresponding vertebra, in this case vertebra seven.[1,2]

Ribs nine through twelve only have one joint (costovertebral) and attach directly to the adjoining vertebra. Rib one has two attachments to the first thoracic vertebra.

EXTERNAL, INNER, AND INNERMOST INTERCOSTAL MUSCLES

There are three layers of intercostal muscles: the external intercostal muscles, which are superficial to the internal intercostal muscles; the internal intercostal muscles, which are inner to the external intercostal muscles; and the innermost intercostal muscles.

External Intercostal Muscles

Origin: Inferior borders of ribs 1–11.[3]
Insertion: Superior borders of ribs 2–12.[3]

General Function/Action: Forced and quiet inhalation. These muscles raise the ribs and expand the chest cavity with inhalation.[3]

Internal Intercostal Muscles

Origin: Ribs 2–12.[3]
Insertion: Ribs 1–11.[3]
General Function/Action: Forced exhalation. These muscles depress the chest cavity and decrease space.[3]

Innermost Intercostal Muscles

Origin: Inferior posterior border of each rib 1–12 (above).[3]
Insertion: Superior posterior border of each rib (below).[3]
General Function/Action: Forced exhalation. These muscles draw in the rib cage.[3]

INTERCOSTAL MUSCLES: WHAT IS THEIR PURPOSE?

The intercostal muscles assist with breathing, oxygen exchange, decompression, stability for the arm, stability for the head, core stability, and prevention of incontinence and prolapse. They also shape your image and help you with performance and sport. Their functions are vital and plentiful, as you will soon start to see!

BREATHING:

A MOST VITAL FUNCTION

The intercostal muscles are used to assist with breathing, both with inhalation and exhalation. Studies show that most people use less and less of their total lung capacity as they age.[4] But this does not have to be the case. Most individuals also never really think about breathing; it's natural right? I would disagree; *breathing has become far from natural for the normal human being. It is not part of our lifestyle to breathe with full capacity and most do not even think about the breath.* Even for the ones who do think about breathing, even for the yogi enthusiast, it's not an in depth thought. Most are all still focused on just the diaphragm for breathing. But it is the whole deep core that allows for breathing. The intercostal muscles are positioned around your lungs and have the ability to lift and compress your ribs/lungs, thus allowing more space for oxygen to fill the lungs and our blood stream.

Normal mechanics of breathing involve pressure changes in the body relative to atmospheric pressure. The breathing system is high pressure chasing low pressure. For the lungs to inflate, the air pressure in your lungs has to be less than the air pressure outside the lungs. This is because air moves from high pressure areas to low pressure areas. At high altitude, the air pressure is lower, therefore making it harder for you to inhale.

In restful breathing, as you inhale, the diaphragm contracts (tightens) and moves downward from a domed position higher in your ribs to more of a flattened position lower in your ribs. This lowering of the diaphragm acts as a vacuum for air to come in. By moving out of the thoracic cavity and into the abdominal cavity, the diaphragm also assists in expanding the lung capacity/volume.

The external intercostal muscles contract, shorten, and move upward and outward, also expanding the lung capacity. The pelvic floor drops and the abdominal cavity expands, further decompressing and assisting with lung capacity/volume and the vacuum effect. With the assistance of these deep core muscles, the lungs become depressurized; the lung cavity pressure becomes lower than the atmospheric pressure, allowing air to flow into the lungs and oxygen exchange to occur.

Where does the inhaled air go? In general, with normal breathing at rest, the lower portion of the chest fills with air laterally (to the sides), anteriorly (to the front), and posteriorly (into the back). Next, the air fills the mid chest and then the upper chest.

As the lungs fill, pressure increases to become higher than atmospheric pressure and exhalation is initiated. The diaphragm goes back up into the thoracic cavity as it relaxes to assist with increased pressure for exhalation. The transverse abdominis compresses and the pelvic floor moves up toward the head, all to naturally assist with exhalation. The internal intercostal muscles contract, moving the ribs down and in. After studying the pelvic floor, transverse abdominis, and multifidi, it should be becoming easier to understand how the deep core works dynamically together as you breathe.

Shockingly, many people do not breathe normally and many lack full breathing and lung capacity. I believe that to have full breathing capacity, you have to optimize your deep core strength, mobility, and coordination. As stated before, as we age, studies show that lung capacity is reduced. I personally believe that this is largely because our lifestyle changes as we age. The body changes due to whatever stresses or lack of stresses we put on it. But does it have to be this way? NO WAY! I have personally expanded my lower intercostal muscles as a pair (left and right) from two centimeters to three inches. Furthermore, many of my patients, from adolescents to eighty-year-olds, have increased their rib expansion no matter their age. Increased intercostal mobility and strength means the potential for increased lung capacity and more oxygen in your lungs and in your blood stream. Vitality!

Why do you need to work on breathing? On one hand, breathing is natural and you will always breathe or you will be dead. On the other hand, you will also choose the path of least resistance and effort. The deep core muscles used for breathing might not be *turned on* or working to their full capacity. You might not be breathing as efficiently or as deeply as you could be. For most people, this is a definite place to optimize function and performance.

INTERCOSTAL MUSCLES AND SHOULDER CONNECTIONS

What if you injure your shoulder due to lifting a heavy or unexpected weight and you "pull a muscle"? The whole shoulder and arm becomes guarded and less used as you attempt to protect this injured area. The tissues and muscles of the shoulder and arm also have connections to the rib cage, either directly or indirectly. In time, these connections may tighten up and your breathing muscles may become restricted, making it harder for you to breathe into the affected area.

Why would you push through tightened, sometimes painful tissue to breathe? You wouldn't! The body chooses to work around this compromised area. It chooses to breathe without effort — the path of least resistance and pain.

Unless you have a good understanding of what has just happened to you or what normal breathing is like, you may never address the issue of the compromised intercostal muscles and all the surrounding tissues. Often the range of motion in the shoulder and intercostal muscles return to a functional state (for movements of day-to-day activities) once the pain goes away; however, the shoulder and the deep core intercostal muscles are often not fully restored to the full potential needed for sport and optimal mechanics. Even if you see a therapist who works on restoring shoulder and arm mechanics, they may neglect the intercostal muscles. A shoulder injury can also move past the intercostal muscles and affect the pelvis, neck, visceral organs, etc., which is beyond the scope of this book.

Just like all the other deep core muscles, the intercostal muscles can turn off and not turn back on again. Or maybe they are *turned on* but not functioning at full capacity. Can you see how easily a shoulder injury could turn these muscles off or decrease the full capacity of lung expansion? At any time in our lives, we can develop poor breathing patterns. It would benefit us all to know what a normal and functional state is and what can happen when things are not normal. In general, most people do not take the time to analyze their breathing. But we need to do that — for sport, life, and health. Many things in our lives can cause improper breathing patterns and directly or indirectly affect our intercostal muscles.

Going back to the example of the shoulder injury, let's say your right shoulder girdle muscles tighten up. Now your ribs feel as though they have a vise on them. The result is that the body will simply bypass the right upper thoracic. The body might compensate by using the shoulder muscles to expand the lungs. With time, the shoulder should heal to some degree, but the motor pathways may not. For example, the pectoralis (chest) muscles and upper trapezius muscle might now be expanding your right thoracic rib cage secondary to the right shoulder injury. This is not ideal, as shoulder mechanics will be disrupted along with the postural and breathing muscles of the right thoracic (the intercostal muscles). Therefore, you will lose optimal performance in both your lungs and shoulders.

In other situations, loss of lung capacity unfolds over time. The decreasing capacity of the shoulder and rib cage may be less obvious. As an example, if you are a mother of a newborn (this is a classic issue, by the way), you may find that you are constantly making the perfect cradle on your chest for both carrying and breastfeeding the baby. In order to make this amazing cradle, your pectoralis, thoracic, and shoulder muscles move into an overall flexed and protracted position. Unfortunately, after a while, you may notice that these muscles do not go back to their lengthened position. The upper thoracic muscles, bones, and tissue get locked into an overall flexed position. Now you are stuck with your rib cage locked into flexion and, potentially, rotation (favoring holding baby to one side can cause the rotation), with tight and dysfunctional intercostal muscles and pectoralis muscles. You may be unable to fully extend without bodywork, tissue mobilization, or the use of specific exercises.

Upper body flexion can also happen from sitting on a bike for a prolonged period of time with protracted shoulders and a rounded back. But at least in this situation the pectoralis and thoracic muscles are symmetrically tight and in a state of overall flexion verses additional rotation from carrying a baby in a one-sided posture. *Pay attention* to the muscles attached to your rib cage and how they have a vise-like effect on the expansion and contraction of your ribs. Furthermore, pay attention to how your body positions can morph you and literally change the way you breathe.

DIRECT TRAUMA

The intercostal muscles may become dysfunctional immediately following motor vehicle accidents, surgeries, illnesses, etc. General lack of use, not exercising and/or moving, can also cause the intercostal muscles to become dysfunctional. All of these situations have the potential to change your posture, your breathing, and ultimately your body's performance. Can you see how these life experiences may change the body's soft tissue (muscle and connective tissues) and the alignment of the skeletal system?

Can you see how a person could continue to lead a normal life while breathing with decreased lung capacity? Most people do not realize that they are lacking lung capacity, rib expansion, and/or intercostal muscle strength because they are not looking and feeling for these changes. The intercostal muscles and the rest of the deep core muscles are not easily seen by the general public, or by the majority of health care professionals. Health care professionals might test your gross leg and arm strength and even isolate specific muscles groups, but how many have said to you, "Wow, your intercostal muscles are really weak!" or "One side of your ribs is not even expanding" or told you that "your intercostal muscles are not even *turned on*"? Start to make positive changes in how you position yourself, heal yourself, and exercise to strengthen your intercostal muscles. SEE the deep core in you!

INTERCOSTAL MUSCLES PROVIDE A STABLE PLATFORM
FOR THE SHOULDER GIRDLE

In my opinion, the intercostal muscles are vital for the shoulder girdle to function properly. The intercostal muscles and ribs act as a platform for the shoulder girdle to sit on. The position at which the scapula sits on the thoracic cage will have effects on the mechanics of the glenohumeral (arm) joint and the scapulothoracic (shoulder blade) joint.

When people start to become weak in their intercostal muscles, it is usually not obvious since there is no pain or notable restrictions. Often, one will feel nothing and see nothing and many times the restrictions are not ever felt at the intercostal muscles. For example, you might feel shoulder pain or a lack of range of motion or strength versus pain or weakness in the intercostal muscles.

Let me share a personal example: Ten plus years ago, I did a lot of rock climbing. I was a 5.10 climber with ease and pushing 5.12s. But at some point my left shoulder was not able to lift me up as well. So, what had happened? The left shoulder felt heavy and weaker with pull-ups. During day-to-day activities, it was fine — but if I did a lot of repetitive lifting during work, it would feel a little tight.

Because I had used the word "heavy" to describe my weakness, a shoulder surgeon gave me an MRI for my cervical region and my head to look for multiple sclerosis. The results were negative. The MRI did point out a herniated disc, which the doctor did not even mention — this I found out later through a different doctor who commented on the MRI results. By the way, many doctors consider herniated discs to be normal. Although herniated discs are normally seen on imaging, they are not a normal result/finding.

What was actually going on with my left shoulder was that my left thoracic spine was collapsing and shifting. There was poor breathing ability and strength in my left intercostal muscles to support my shoulder girdle. It took me years to be able to produce this self-diagnosis that now seems so simple. I was not breathing correctly and my intercostal muscles were weak and tight. My scapulothoracic muscles were also being constricted and that too was restricting my breathing.

Now I know that the intercostal muscles are a stable platform for the shoulder girdle. I feel this quite strongly, especially since I know what it felt like to have a strong base for my shoulder (intercostal strength and alignment), then not to have that strength, and finally for it to return with due diligence again. This was SO REJU-VENATING! Words cannot adequately explain my relief.

Other classical conditions where the intercostal muscles are weak or tight and therefore affect the position of the shoulder girdle include kyphosis, scoliosis, thoracic or lumbar shifts, broken ribs, lobectomies (removal of lobes of lung), poor rib alignment, thoracic injuries, and medical diagnoses that restrict normal mechanics of the rib cage and intercostal muscles.

Mary is an amazing physical therapist and a true specialist in breathing. She has a true gift and passion for helping individuals, specifically children, with significant postural and breathing impairments. Her soda pop can theory is used to help explain the mechanics of breathing and postural support, stability, and trunk control.[5] Pressure — the breath — assists to keep the body upright and stable. The muscles of the trunk also help to assist us in breathing. As Mary likes to say, "If you can't breathe, you can't function."[5]

According to the soda pop can theory, the deep core is a pressure system much like a soft drink can. The glottis (the opening between the vocal folds) is the top of the can, where you open it. The upper half of the soda pop can is the rib cage. At the center of the can, there is a flexible but mobile platform — the diaphragm. Below the diaphragm is the fluid–filled stomach encased by the transverse abdominis. The bottom of the can is your pelvic floor.

Unlike a soda pop can, your deep core is dynamic because it can move. The opening (glottis) can open and close, the top part (lungs) can expand and shorten on all planes, the center (diaphragm) can rise and lower, expand and contract, the abdominals can expand

and shorten, and the pelvic floor can rise and lower, open and close. This system can be very strong, like an unopened soda pop can.

Now imagine both ends of the system closed (the glottis and the pelvic floor contracted), trapping the pressure, just like an unopened can. It is very difficult to crush an unopened can compared to an open can. We use this strength if we need stability. For example, if we are being pushed, we might contract the pelvic floor and glottis to become more stable. A gymnast is a good example of an athlete who might need this type of stability. When a gymnast is constantly holding a position, they are holding their breath momentarily for increased support.

OUR INTERNAL PRESSURE SYSTEM: DISEASED

Let's look at this pressure system, in essence our deep core, and how it can be affected. As an example, emphysema is a disease that affects the alveoli (multiple small air sacs) in the lungs. The alveoli allow oxygen to enter and carbon dioxide to exit the blood during breathing. Emphysema can be caused by smoking (cigarettes and marijuana), inhalation of chemical fumes or dust, air pollution, and less commonly by a lack of protein. The little air sacs weaken and rupture, creating one big air sac with less overall circumference and therefore less oxygen exchange sites into the surrounding capillaries. The lack of these precious oxygen exchange sites is, in essence, lack of oxygen to our cells.

Emphysema is described as a chronic obstructive pulmonary disease. With less oxygen exchange, our body is holding more stagnant oxygen in the lungs and carbon dioxide in the blood. This creates an obstruction. It becomes harder for the body to refill with fresh oxygen and expel carbon dioxide. When oxygen levels are low and there is a high carbon dioxide level in the body, the body's tissues suffer. This is detrimental to cardio activities such as running, swimming, biking, walking, and just day-to-day activities. Respiratory failure can occur when the disease is severe. People with emphysema can benefit from a concerted strengthening of the deep core muscles in order to help combat their dysfunctional alveoli. Strengthening the deep core will maximize the number of oxygen exchange sites that are available.

It is important to maximize the mobility and strength of your intercostal muscles to improve your lung function, not only to prevent and treat diseases, but also to improve your performance. The same little techniques that physical therapists and medical professionals use to keep people alive from deadly diseases can also be used by athletes to get an edge in their sport. Activating the deep core is one of these techniques.

COILING AND RECOILING OF THE RIBS
FOR OXYGEN EXCHANGE

If your ribs are not able to open and close to full range, there is less space for air to come and go. There is also less potential for oxygen exchange in the lungs. For this reason, your intercostal muscles should be trained to reach their full range in both expansion and shortening.

LACK OF MOBILITY IN THE RIB CAGE
AND THE EFFECT AT THE PELVIC FLOOR

Lack of mobility in the rib cage can affect the pelvic floor and abdominals. It will affect the bottom half of your soda pop can. With less expansion of the ribs with inhalation, pressure will increase at the next tissue that will move, which is your lower half, the abdominals and pelvic floor. What if your ribs do not expand with a sneeze? The lungs normally naturally expand in response to this force. If the ribs are restricted, pressure will build at your abdominals and pelvic floor, which often leads to incontinence and/or prolapse.

LACK OF RIB EXPANSION: COULD IT CONTRIBUTE TO
RIB FRACTURES WITH A COMMON COLD?

The pressure of a sneeze or cough can be so strong that it even fractures ribs. This is known to happen with medical diagnoses such as osteoporosis, osteopenia, brittle bone disease, and bone cancer. However, studies also show that it can happen with normal, healthy bone density.[6] I believe that this happens when there is a lack of flexibility in the intercostal muscles — a lack of ability to coil and recoil — along with restricted fascia of the ribs. Research demonstrates that fascia is stronger than steel. Interestingly, I had a patient with a titanium rod within their femur that was found broken on imaging. How did this happen? My guess is that tight fibrotic fascia contraction broke the rod. Yes, fascia can contract. The intercostal muscles can be tight and restrictive, also leaving the bone at risk for breaking and/or the muscle tissue at risk for tearing rather than just stretching with the increased pressure.

I have used this force to mobilize my tight thoracic region; when I sneeze or cough, I will sometimes direct this force to the intercostal muscles. I do this with intention, positioning, and thoughtful activation of the core. This obviously has to be done with caution, and I would not necessarily recommend it.

INTERCOSTAL MUSCLES:

OUR NATURAL DECOMPRESSION SYSTEM

The intercostal muscles, along with the rest of the deep core, are an essential part of our natural decompression system. The intercostal muscles are able to help lift the ribs and indirectly decompress the vertebrae, thereby decreasing stress at the joints. With the vertebrae decompressed, blood flow is able to provide healthy nutrients to the joint spaces, specifically the vertebral discs and joints, but also to compressed muscle and fascia tissue. Space is being created with the breath. There is a constant coil and recoil, the same coil and recoil one should desire with their diaphragm, pelvic floor, and transverse abdominis.

The natural compression and decompression of the ribs and chest allows for a natural decompression of the spine. Think about it: our natural, built-in decompression system. Our body is amazing. All we have to do is maximize our breathing and we have a built-in traction system to take pressure off of our joints and tissues.

The compression forces that we fight every day include natural gravity, our own body weight, our own cellular restrictions (muscle, fascia, bone), and the weight that we carry physically, emotionally, and mentally. Yes, *mentally and emotionally.* The more I work with patients, the more emotions of all kinds I find in muscle and fascia. Some of the biggest releases happen in the body's tissues when emotions are also released. Often these releases are accompanied by crying, yelling, facial expressions, and/or physical movements. Our emotions are definitely imprinted onto our muscles. Muscles and tissues have memory and they talk and express themselves to the rest of the body (this is a topic for another book, but something I want you to know is real).

ROTATION: AN IMPORTANT FUNCTION OF THE INTERCOSTAL MUSCLES AND THORACIC VERTEBRAE

Intercostal muscles that are functioning normally, with strength and mobility, allow for a healthy state of rotation for both life and sport. Rotation is important for normal day-to-day movement and it is essential for athletes. For example, when you are running, you want your thoracic rib cage to move you. You do not want to run with a stiff thoracic spine, nor do you want to take the rotation from elsewhere (pelvis, shoulders). Not only are your intercostal muscles constantly decompressing your spine, they are also winding you up and propelling you with every rotation.

I would go further and argue that control of air is also providing rotation when you are running. Have you really thought about *where* the air you inhale while running is positioning itself within your body? I believe that each time you swing your right arm forward, your rib cage responds by expanding more anteriorly on the right and posteriorly on the left, and vice versa when you swing your left arm. Think about it: your air directing your rotation through the biomechanics of running.

Once I was working with an elderly patient who was struggling to breath. She was in her last days of life. She was breathing in an interesting pattern, very interesting! AMAZING ACTUALLY! She would breathe into her left front and right back, and then into her right front and left back simultaneously. It was like her rib cage was walking. This got me thinking — maybe uncomfortable breathing when learning how to run or swim is just the body learning where to put the air most effectively? Maybe this woman was using her ribs most efficiently to assist her with functional mobility, with survival. It is likely she was using her ribs to assist her with walking.

I do believe every sport and functional task requires a different breathing pattern for efficiency; maximizing these skills would, in essence, improve performance. Why not start with at least being able to identify the breathing muscles? Identify your deep core, and then maximize the range of motion and strength within the deep core to assist you with your sport and functional demands. Starting with full or near full capacity on inhale and exhale at all levels of your intercostal muscles optimizes the potential to get air where we need it for sport and life so we have the strength and mobility to meet our physical demands, needs, and wants.

On the flip side, use sports to gain an edge in your intercostal muscle strength. Certain sports and activities, such as swimming, can assist with increasing lung capacity and intercostal muscle strength and mobility to enhance your day-to-day life.

LESSONS FROM NATURE

Let nature prevail the secrets: Once I was attempting to fly-fish with my fiancé, now husband, in Belize. We had rented a sit-on-top kayak and taken it to a more remote island just off of Caye Caulker. We had the place all to ourselves, or so we thought. While my husband was watching the fish avoid his bait, I saw a small bushy tree branch move violently and what looked like a log floating in the water. I said to my husband, "I think that log is a crocodile. Look at that branch move!" He shook his head and said it was just a log. The "log" moved quite a bit, further down the creek that separated the small island. I knew that it was a crocodile (Figure 5.4).

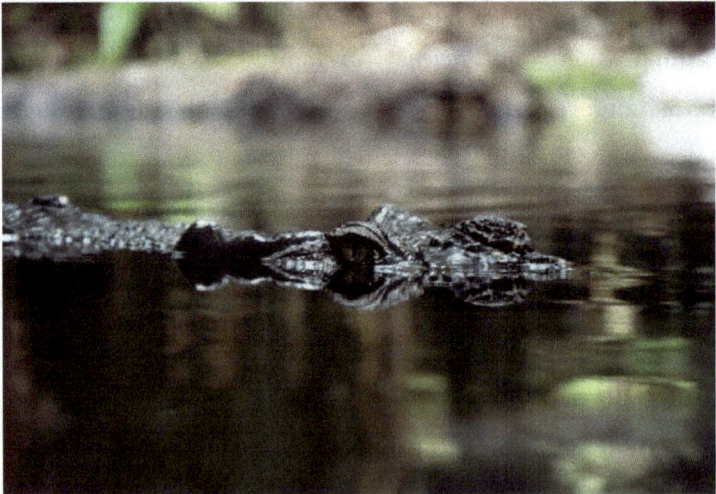

Figure 5.4. A sneaky creature.
From Rehoboth foto/*Shutterstock.com.*

When we returned the next day, the crocodile was easily visible and very close to the shore where we had planned to go fishing. My husband saw it clearly and happily agreed that we should not fish there that day. I began to wonder how these creatures could slink along so silently and move so stealthily, since on the first day it was only about sixty feet from us and I had really concentrated on it while I was attempting to fish.

When I got back to the States, I researched crocodiles and alligators. I learned that alligators use their lungs to move without making a ripple. They are sneaky and silent. Alligators are able to use their breath to move by expanding one lung, then the other. It is also interesting how they position the air in their lungs when they dive in and out of the water and roll.[7] Alligators use their diaphragm, pelvic, abdominal, and rib musculature to shift their lungs like internal flotation devices.[8]

THINK ABOUT YOUR INTERCOSTAL MUSCLES WITH SWIMMING

What do we do with our own intercostal muscles when swimming? Let's think about the act of swimming the front crawl. You need thoracic rotation to propel yourself through the water and to take breaths. Imagine if you were able to have full rotation in your thoracic rib cage and intercostal muscles — breathing to each side could become less of an effort.

Breathing on only one side while swimming can cause intercostal muscles and rib mobility to become restricted. Asymmetrical rotation can also lead to swimming in a non-straight line. Whenever you primarily use just one side of your body for breathing, muscular imbalances can occur throughout the body.

INTERCOSTAL MUSCLES: ALIGNMENT AND SO ON

If your body is bilaterally or unilaterally weak at the intercostal muscles, it could lead to poor alignment. As an example, if the intercostal muscles are shortened at multiple levels and stuck in a flexed position, the spine will be bent over. A misaligned spine is like a misaligned car — you will not function properly or reliably. The car might drive crookedly down the road, just like an out-of-alignment human might walk circuitously. Or your core might not be able to expend energy as efficiently since it is forced to bypass several muscles that are not firing correctly due to poor alignment. If the intercostal muscles become dysfunctional, they fail at their ability to do their job of maintaining alignment, strength, stability, mobility, posture, breathing, circulation, and image.

The intercostal muscles indirectly connect to the spine via the ribs. As a result, if the intercostal muscles are restricted, then the ribs and vertebrae can also become restricted. If your breath is restricted in one area, it usually translates to a restriction at that same vertebral level. You can use your intercostal muscles to mobilize and decompress your spine by turning the intercostals back on and/or increasing their strength and mobility. Use your intercostal muscles to assist with re-aligning and restoring mobility at a vertebral level.

The intercostal muscles can be stuck in any position: rotated, flexed, extended, shifted, and/or twisted. We need to free them! Breathe with effort, focus, and force — use your muscles to assist you!

INTERCOSTAL MUSCLES SHAPE YOU

Intercostal muscles are a sign of strength and power. They really have the ability to shape your torso. Just look at a drawing of your favorite superhero; most have a massive chest, and this is not their chest musculature (pectoralis major and minor) that the artist is portraying. This is their intercostal muscles, and really the whole deep core working as a well designed dynamic pressure system. When the superhero displays signs of increased power, their thoracic wall expands and puffs outward. This is a classic way of expressing something that everyone relates to visually. The intercostal muscles lengthen and the lungs fill with air — POWER!

Without the ability to expand your ribs with the use of the deep core, more so the intercostals, the body will be challenged to get air and take form! The intercostals, like all of the deep core muscles, help to shape your torso's architecture and image.

POSTURE IN SPORT

Posture and alignment ARE EVERYTHING IN SPORT. The deep core is the framework for your posture. Mobility and strength at your pelvic floor, transverse abdominis, multifidi, intercostal muscles, and diaphragm will enhance your performance. A strong and mobile framework is ideal. A simple way to correct your posture is not to squeeze your shoulder blades back, but rather to fully inhale and exhale using your intercostals.

Your body functions best when it is aligned and in good posture. When the deep core is not *turned on,* you will struggle for activation and strength throughout your body. Posture, alignment, mobility, and strength are what the deep core has to offer. These components will affect agility, timing, and efficient motor strategies.

HOW DO YOU KNOW IF YOUR INTERCOSTAL MUSCLES ARE *TURNED ON?*

Circumferential Measurements

Measuring your rib cage is one way of identifying if your intercostal muscles are turned on and have some mobility. Measuring can give general information about a specific area of your rib cage. Try measuring your lower, mid, and upper costal expansion circumferentially as described below.

Lower Intercostal Expansion: Find your xiphoid process at the bottom of your sternum (see Figure 5.3). Measure halfway between your xiphoid process and your umbilicus (belly button). Wrap a flexible measuring tape around yourself at that level. Throughout the measuring process, make sure you are sitting or standing with good posture. Fully exhale and think, "Make yourself as small as possible around your lower ribs on all sides of the body," while taking that measurement. Then fully inhale and think, "Make yourself as big as possible in your lower ribs," and take that measurement. The difference between the two measurements is the rib expansion at your lower intercostal muscles.

Table 5.1. Mean circumferential rib expansion at the fourth intercostal space by sex and age. Adapted from Moll et al.[9]

Age (years)	Female mean (cm)	Male mean (cm)
15–24	5.55	7.01
25–34	5.46	7.37
35–44	4.57	6.56
45–54	4.82	6.00
55–64	3.77	5.51
65–74	3.76	4.00
75 and up	2.45	2.81

Middle Intercostal Expansion: Find your fourth intercostal space. This space is approximately at your nipple line depending on the amount of breast tissue. Another way to find the fourth intercostal space is to identify the sternal angle below the manubrium and go laterally — you will hit the second rib (see Figure 5.3). Below the second rib is your second intercostal space. Count down from there to find the fourth intercostal space. Again, maintain good posture while sitting or standing. Wrap a flexible tape around your body at the level of the fourth intercostal space. Maximally exhale, "Make your chest as small as possible," and take that measurement. Then maximally inhale, "Make your chest as big as possible on all sides of the body," and take that measurement. The difference between these two measurements is the rib expansion at your middle intercostal muscles (see Table 5.1).

Upper Intercostal Expansion: Wrap a flexible tape around your body below your armpit while maintaining good posture. Fully exhale and think, "Make your upper chest as small as possible." Take your measurement. Then inhale, "Make your upper chest as big as possible," and take that measurement. The difference between the measurements is the upper thoracic rib expansion at your upper intercostal muscles.

NOTE: Ideally the middle intercostal expansion measurements should be taken by a second person while your arms are overhead. To reflexively increase expansion at any measured level of circumference, you can sniff at the presumed end range of inhalation. Remember, sometimes weakness is just on one side. You might be asymmetrical in your expansion/strength. Therefore, you can measure just one side at a time; measure from your backbone to the center of your chest on the right and then the left. A second person might be nice for this.

Look and Feel for Expansion and Decompression

Expansion in the front, back, and sides of your rib cage is a sign that your intercostal muscles are *turned on*. Start by checking the front lower ribs. Stand in front of a mirror with your shirt off and put the palms of your hands over your upper abdominal muscles and lower ribs on the front of your body, just below your sternum ideally. Maximally exhale and feel for your ribs to go down towards your spine. Then maximally inhale; are you able to see or feel a rise of your ribs at this level?

Now move your palms to the sides of your lower intercostal muscles, at the same level of your torso. Assess to see whether your ribs are expanding and decompressing. Again, maximally exhale and feel for the ribs moving inward. Then fully inhale and assess for expansion laterally (on the sides of your lower intercostal muscles).

Finally, at the same level of your torso, wrap your thumb and/or hand to the back of your lower ribs. Feel for the ribs to move inwards with maximal exhalation and outward with inhalation.

Are you able to breathe in all directions and spaces of your rib cage with full inhalation and exhalation? Are your sides symmetrical? Do the same assessments at mid chest (at your fourth intercostal space) and then at your upper chest. If you do notice lack of mobility, this is a sign that your intercostal muscles are weak, tight, or dysfunctional in some way.

Grab a partner for this test. Have your partner attempt to resist you from raising your arm. Specifically, have them lightly resist your arm movement past shoulder height. With your other arm, try to touch your ribs and FEEL if there is any activation of the intercostal muscles between the ribs. Also feel between the ribs for muscle tone. Look and feel if your body bends to either side in the spine while attempting to resist your partner. Is the spine collapsing or giving way with resistance? If so, the intercostals could be failing to support resistance. If the spine collapses, it is a sign that the thoracic intercostal muscles are weak. It is also a sign of weakness if you do not feel your intercostal muscles contract between your ribs.

HOW CAN YOU *TURN ON* THE INTERCOSTAL MUSCLES?

There are endless ways to *turn on* the intercostal muscles. Try some of the below:

Sniffs

Take three quick sniffs through the nose, then two slower, longer sniffs, and finally one long sniff. Then relax and let the body reflexively recoil to exhale. Repeat these actions and attempt to make each sniff longer. The focus here is on your lower intercostal muscles and diaphragm. I like to think of sniffs as a way to reflexively sneak some more air in.

Forced Inhalation

Take a deep breath in through your nose or mouth. Bring your inhalation to end range. Like superman, try to puff out your entire rib cage to end range. Then, when you think you are at end range, try to push past any muscular or fascial restrictions with increased inhalation. You can actually use your breath to mobilize your ribs and intercostal muscles, and indirectly your vertebrae and muscles throughout your torso.

Forced Exhalation

Exhale to end range. Think of using your intercostal muscles to assist in this process. Bring your ribs inward as far as you are able using your intercostal muscles, abdominal muscles, and pelvic floor. Then relax and reflexively inhale.

Tummy Time

Lying on your back, place an object on your upper tummy and try to get it to move as high as you can with inhalation and as low as you can with exhalation. The focus here is on the lower intercostal muscles and diaphragm on both the posterior and anterior plane. Increase lateral expansion of your lower ribs by moving your arms away from your sides and focusing on bringing air to the sides of your lower ribs.

Lateral Mobility and Strength of Intercostal Muscles

Lie on your left side. Place your right hand on your right lower ribs and inhale. Inhale to end range lateral rib expansion and hold your ribs at end range expansion for five seconds. After five seconds, keep the ribs stationary but exhale as much air as you can without your ribs moving from the elevated position. Then forcefully exhale with the intercostals, transverse abdominis, and pelvic floor muscles. Bring the ribs inwards toward the center of your body. Relax. Relax initially for at least ten seconds between reps with this exercise. Then repeat on the other side. This exercise demonstrates that the intercostals can be a stabilizer versus just a breathing muscle. Note that you could exhale while keeping the ribs elevated.

The Power of Intention

The power of intention is important with all deep core exercises. The previous exercises require focus and thought, not just movement. Try to envision the intercostal muscles working along with all the deep core muscles. Start to see the harmony between the deep core muscles.

Intentional Breathing with Lifting Weights

When lifting weights, focus on breathing to expand the lungs. Do this with lengthening movements. For example, with raising your arms up for overhead presses, take a deep breath in while lifting the weights up and forcefully exhale when bringing them down.

Add Breath to Your Daily Movements

Intentionally exaggerate inhalation while reaching into your higher cupboards. Think about expanding your lungs while reaching your arms up. When bringing your arms down from the cupboard, as an example, exhale and let your muscles recoil. When turning to grab something, use the breath to assist with the rotation of your ribs and to increase the space between the ribs while rotating your thoracic spine. When yawning, focus on excessive breathing into your ribs, puffing your rib cage out on all sides. When just sitting at your desk, do some deep breaths frequently throughout the day.

Use Your Breath to Shape You

Remember, your breath shapes you! When going about your day, focus on your posture — just breathe deeply into your ribs. This is a sneaky way to correct your posture. Eventually these muscles will have more mobility with inhalation and exhalation and naturally be working for you with every breath to hold your posture and stability. This is much better than simple squeezing your shoulder blades together when "correcting posture." Overly squeezing the shoulder blades together often actually blocks the backside of the thoracic rib cage from fully expanding. I like to cue patients to lengthen their chest on the frontal plane to correct shoulder girdle position.

Position Matters

There are certain positions that will assist in addressing your upper, middle, and lower intercostal muscles. Certain positions can also assist with right and left intercostal muscles.

You can position your arms to activate different areas of your intercostal muscles/ribs. It is good to know how to isolate your weak areas to make them stronger, if you know where they are. This is why we separate the intercostal muscles into three sections (upper, middle, lower) and left and right, front and back. If your left side is weak, for example, block your right side by putting your hand or arm at your right side or lying on your right side. Then lift your left arm over your head to allow air to more easily enter into the left side. If you want to make it harder for your left lateral side, you could use a band to add resistance. You could also use the force of your hand as a form of resistance. External perturbation is another technique used to activate the deep core muscles and provide resistance. Perturbation involves applying unanticipated forces to disturb postural control.

Gaze: The Power of the Eyes

Gaze assists with exhalation and inhalation. Upward gaze assists with inhalation. Downward gaze assists with exhalation.

Magic Fingers

You can use the positioning of just your fingers to assist with directing your breath within your chest. I don't know why this works. I'm assuming these are primal movements we did as monkeys or in past generations.

- Upper Chest: Make a fist with thumb enclosed by the other four fingers.
- Middle Chest: Make a fist with thumb over fist.
- Lower Chest: Form a circle with thumb and next two fingers and fully lengthen the pinky and the ring finger.

Interestingly, it does not matter where your hands are. Rather, the positioning of your digits seems to direct the air to the desired locations. You can add these finger positions to intercostal exercises or to cardiovascular activity.

Superman

Simply try to puff your chest out the way superheroes are commonly portrayed in comic books. Breathe into your chest or wherever in your intercostal muscles you would like to focus. Breathe powerfully and with intent, pushing past fascia and muscle restrictions. Use the breathing muscles to expand your rib cage. With this expansion, you are not only assisting in activation and strengthening of the intercostals; but also with mobility, stretching, and releasing tight tissues.

Focus on Inhalation Strength: Imagine that you are trying to take a dent out of your chest. Push the air into the weakened intercostal muscles. Feel for the muscle and fascia to stretch. Feel for the ribs to expand. Rest for ten to thirty seconds following each repetition. Repeat five to ten times.

Focus on Exhalation Strength: Try to fully and forcefully exhale all air from your lungs. Then reflexively or forcefully inhale. Rest for ten to thirty seconds following each repetition. Repeat five to ten times.

Isometric Strengthening at End Ranges

Holding at End Range Inhale: Take a deep breath in. When you get as much in as you can, push more air in. Hold air in and ribs out for one to ten seconds and then exhale. Progress to ten-second holds, making sure to take ten- to thirty-second rests between repetitions.

Holding at End Range Exhalation: Push all of the air out of your lungs. When you think you cannot push any more air out, use your pelvic floor, abdominals, and intercostal muscles to push more air out. Hold for one to ten seconds. Then happily breathe in again. Progress to ten-second holds, making sure to take ten- to thirty-second rests between repetitions.

Maximize Your End Range Mobility and Strength

Inhalation Muscles and End Range Inhalation: Inhale to end range over a six-second span, then exhale over a four-second span. Progress by increasing inhalation count and/or decreasing exhalation count.

The body will ask the intercostal muscles to push through restrictions at the intercostal muscles themselves or at fascia, bone, and muscle. The body will choose to breath.

Exhalation Muscles and End Range Exhalation: Getting air out of the lungs is also important. Remember that the lungs need to inflate and deflate. Sometimes the ribs can get stuck in an outward position. This could indicate that the exhalation muscles are weak and/or restricted. Inhale to end range for two seconds, exhale for four seconds. Progress by increasing exhalation time relative to inhalation time.

Coordination

Moving Air Slowly: Inhale for three seconds and exhale for three seconds. Progress seconds of inhalation and exhalation.

Moving Air Quickly: Attempt to expel air out of the lungs quickly. Try for more volume in less time. Attempt to inhale air into the lungs quickly. Try for more volume in less time.

Yoga

Breathe with your deep core for all poses and transitions. Focus on intention, mobility, flexibility, and strength in your deep core muscles and associated joints. Use your deep core to draw in more air. Use the air and muscles TO MAKE MORE MOVEMENT AND FLEXI-BILITY. Breathe to actually stretch the tissue, specifically the torso.

Use the power of your deep core strength to draw in the air and the pressure of the air to manipulate obstructed areas. Imagine that you are trying to take a dent out of your ribs or lungs. Or imagine that your lungs are an air mattress and you are trying to get the creases out. The creases in your lungs can be viewed as tight restrictions of muscle or fascia or even bone. All yoga poses will affect different areas of your lungs. Focus on where restrictions are felt.

Singing

Holding notes for an extended time can strengthen the breathing muscles. Singers have many techniques to improve their breathing power.

Intent Matters! Always! Really!

Think urgent, forceful, with effort for your intercostal muscles to activate fully. Make your breath count.

Command Your Body

Command yourself or others loudly to get the intercostal muscles firing: "BREATHE! DEEPER! DEEPER! MORE! FIND MORE!" Yell. Speak to your body: "MORE! FIND MORE SPACE! CREATE THE SPACE! FEEL THE STRETCH BOTH INSIDE THE RIBS AND OUTSIDE! BREATHE PAST YOUR CURRENT MUSCLE AND FASCIAL RESTRICTIONS — STRETCH YOUR LIMITS

— STRETCH YOUR BOUNDARIES!" A little space can be all the body needs for a good self-release! The core can provide.

Who Doesn't Like a Toy?

- "The Breather" is a device that adds resistance (at different levels) with both inhalation and exhalation.[10]
- The AMEO Powerbreather Lap Snorkel can be used with swimming.[11]
- A spirometer measures the volume of air with inhalation and exhalation.
- Commercial-grade hyperbaric chambers are sparsely offered at recovery or wellness centers throughout the US.

Incorporate the Intercostal Muscles into Your Sport

- Take less breaths with swimming, breathing every four to six versus one to two strokes.
- Get a snorkel for swimming, ideally the Powerbreather.
- While running, focus on rib expansion. Focus on multiple levels (upper, middle, lower) and on all sides while on the run.
- While biking, focus on posture and the intercostal muscles, again considering all levels and sides.

REFERENCES

1. Netter FH. *Atlas of Human Anatomy*. 7th ed. Elsevier; 2018.
2. Jones O. The ribs. TeachMe Anatomy. March 30, 2025. Accessed

April 12, 2025. https://teachmeanatomy.info/thorax/bones/ribcage/

3.   The Healthline Editorial Team. Intercostal muscles. Healthline. January 22, 2018. https://www.healthline.com/human-body-maps/intercostal-muscles

4.   Sharp JT, Beard GA, Sunga M, et al. The rib cage in normal and emphysematous subjects: a roentgenographic approach. *Journal of Applied Physiology.* 1986;61:2050-9. doi:10.1152/jappl.1986.61.6.2050

5.   Massery M. Musculoskeletal and neuromuscular interventions: a physical approach to cystic fibrosis. *Journal of Royal Society of Medicine.* 2005;98:55-66.

6.   Hanak V, Hartman TE, Ryu JH. Cough-induced rib fractures. *Mayo Clinic Proceedings.* 2005;80:879-82. doi:10.4065/80.7.879

7.   Yong E. Stealthy alligators dive, rise and roll by moving their lungs. National Geographic. March 14, 2008. Accessed April 12, 2025. https://www.nationalgeographic.com/science/article/stealthy-alligators-dive-rise-and-roll-by-moving-their-lungs

8.   University of Utah. Alligators muscles move lungs around for sneaky maneuvers in water. ScienceDaily. March 14, 2008. Accessed April 12, 2025. https://www.sciencedaily.com/releases/2008/03/080313124451.htm

9.   Moll JM, Wright V. An objective clinical study of chest expansion. *Annals of the Rheumatic Diseases.* 1972;31:1-8. doi:10.1136/ard.31.1.1

10. The Breather. Accessed April 12, 2025. https://www.thebreather.com.au

11. AMEO Watersports. Accessed April 12, 2025. https://www.powerbreather.com/en/

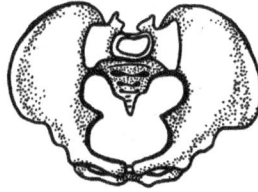

DIAPHRAGM

The diaphragm is two to four millimeters thick.[1] At rest, it is like a hollow dome or a tent in the middle of your torso (Figure 6.1). With full contraction, it moves down in your ribs to your abdominals and flattens out. The diaphragm separates the thoracic and abdominal cavities and contents from one another. Interestingly, it domes higher on the right than on the left to make room for the heart. Due to this difference in heights, the diaphragm at rest actually looks like two domes, versus one big dome as it is often described. The diaphragm spans ribs eight through ten and lumbar vertebrae levels one through three.

The diaphragm is a very integrated muscle. It has numerous fascial, ligamentous, muscle, visceral, nervous, and vascular connections throughout the entire body from the cranium to the pelvis.[1]

With inhalation, the diaphragm contracts concentrically (shortens) and moves down and outward in the rib cage and pushes into the abdominal cavity. When the diaphragm moves down, the lower ribs expand in all directions: left, right, back, and front. Oxygen fills the lungs at the lower lobes, followed by the mid thoracic region, and then the upper lobes of the lungs. With exhalation, the diaphragm moves back up into the rib cage (Figure 6.2).

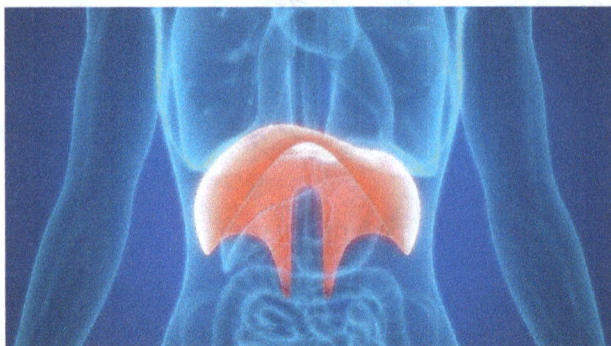

Figure 6.1. The diaphragm.
From Magic mine/*Shutterstock.com.*

Movement of the diaphragm spans a vast majority of your torso. One research study of sixteen healthy subjects with a mean age of thirty-one years demonstrated this.[2] The average amplitude of inferior–superior (up and down) movement of the diaphragm apex during tidal breathing was 27.3 millimeters. During active voluntary movement with breath-holding, the average amplitude was 32.5 millimeters inferior–superior.[2]

When the diaphragm moves down in the torso, it also expands outward and anatomically to all sides of the body, front, back, left, and right. Normal outward expansion of the diaphragm was measured in this study as 39 millimeters with restful breathing and 45.5 millimeters with voluntary breath-holding at the costophrenic angle.[2] The costophrenic angle is where the diaphragm meets the ribs. Interestingly, the diaphragm is working not just at rest automatically, but voluntarily unrelated to a breathing task.[3] The diaphragm is not just functioning for breathing!

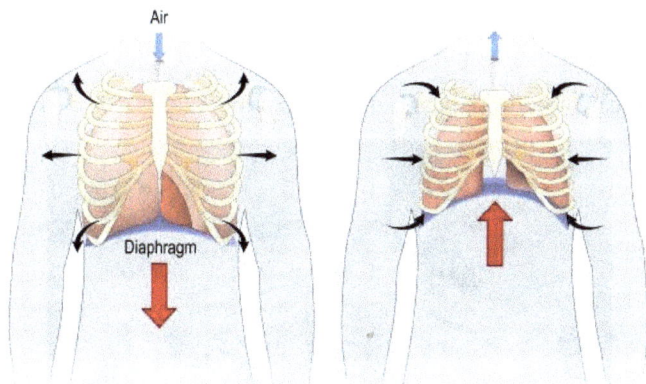

Figure 6.2. Movement of the diaphragm during breathing. Adapted from Designua/*Shutterstock.com.*

THE DIAPHRAGM AS TWO MUSCLES

Scientists are suggesting that the diaphragm be viewed, anatomically and functionally, as two separate muscles that work in synchrony.[4-6] The costal diaphragm is on the outskirts of the body and the crural diaphragm is more central to the core. The crural diaphragm is anatomically different in that it is thicker with more muscle bulk and more isolated to the backside of the body where it attaches to the vertebrae of the spine.[6] We will see how these two muscles have different jobs but work in tandem.

WHO SHOULD CARE ABOUT THE DIAPHRAGM?

An ill-functioning diaphragm can cause many problems, including troubled breathing, asthma or anxiety, difficulty sleeping, stability or balance problems, low back pain, incontinence, and/or digestion disruptions such as GERD. These are just a few of the problems that a dysfunctional diaphragm can set in motion. For these reasons, *we all* need to care about the health of our diaphragm.

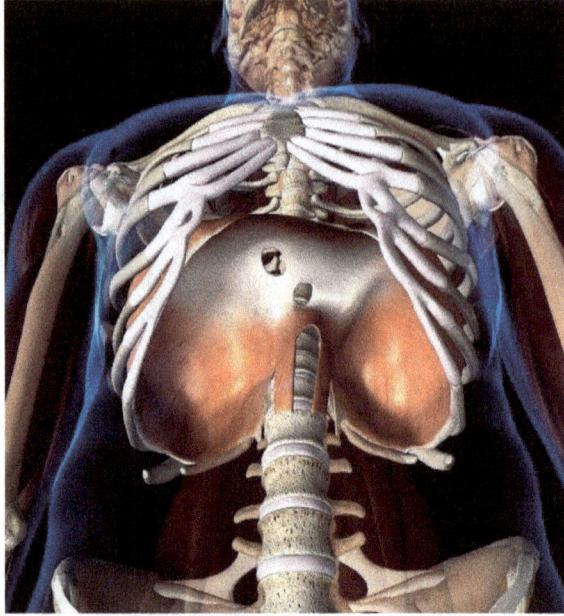

Figure 6.3. The diaphragm is well connected.
From Hank Grebe/*Shutterstock.com.*

HOW THE DIAPHRAGM IS CONNECTED

Origin and Insertion: Not so clear, as the diaphragm is so connected! For identifying purposes, the general origin and insertions are at the sternum, ribs, and lumbar spine (see Figure 6.3).

More on Connections and Insertions: Xiphoid process of the sternum to the same vertebral level of thoracic spine, T8–T9.[1] Ribs six through twelve, inferiorly and laterally.[1,7] Lumbar spinal vertebrae at levels one through three (plus corresponding intervertebral discs).[7] Lumbar portion of the anterior longitudinal ligament (which runs in front of the vertebrae of the entire spine) via the crural legs of the diaphragm.[7] Medial arcuate ligament (which arches over the psoas major) at L1–L2.[7,8] Lateral arcuate ligaments of quadratus lumborum (which pass over the upper part of the quadratus lumborum muscle and under the diaphragm).[7,8]

Action: Contracts outward and downward with inhalation.

INTERESTING ANATOMICAL FEATURES OF THE DIAPHRAGM

Crucs or Legs of the Diaphragm

Two tendinous structures stemming from the diaphragm that connect onto the vertebrae at levels L1-4.[7,8]

Three Major Openings within the Diaphragm

- Vena caval foramen: The inferior vena cava passes through this hole to bring deoxygenated blood back to the heart from the lower body at level T8.[7]
- Esophageal hiatus: This is where the esophagus connects to the stomach at level T10.[7]
- Aortic hiatus: This opening allows the aortic artery to supply oxygenated blood to the lower core and legs at level T12.[7]

The diaphragmatic ligaments are structures that connect the diaphragm to the surrounding organs:

- Phrenopericardial ligament: Connects the diaphragm to the heart.[1]
- Phrenicoesophageal ligament: Connects the diaphragm to the esophagus.[1]
- Phrenicocolic ligament: Connects the diaphragm to the right ascending colon.[1]
- Ligament of Treitz: A series of muscular tracts that begin in the right crus of the diaphragm and go to the duodenojejunal angle.[1,9]

Wait, did you see that? *Look* at all those connections. The diaphragm connects to multiple structures: muscles, vertebrae, discs, ribs, the xiphoid process of your sternum, and to many organs via ligaments.

WHAT IS THE FUNCTION OF THE DIAPHRAGM?

The diaphragm is the primary muscle involved in active inspiration, however it DOES MUCH MORE. The anatomical position and structure of the diaphragm give rise to multiple functions besides breathing, including assistance with posture and stabilization, assistance in maintaining continence of bowel and bladder, assistance in evacuation of bowel and urine, assistance with prevention of GERD, assistance with digestion, and circulation. When studying the anatomy of the diaphragm and its multiple attachments, it is not surprising that it has so many functions.

The diaphragm is primarily a breathing muscle, obviously. However, is your diaphragm *turned on*? Is it working for you? Is it working with full potential?

Most would agree that breathing is the diaphragm's most important function. The lungs cannot contract on their own; it is the deep core muscles that assist in maintaining and initiating this vital function! The diaphragm helps with getting oxygen to your lungs and eventually to your tissues for survival, function, life itself, and SPORT.

The costal muscle of the diaphragm contracts and lowers towards the abdominal region while the lung pressure decreases and the lung volume increases. This allows air to enter the lungs with inhalation, as the high pressure of the air chases the low pressure of the lungs, allowing oxygen exchange. During relaxed breathing, there is passive recoil of the diaphragm, which domes back up into the lungs with exhalation. It is the abdominal muscle contracting that increases pressure and the eccentric contraction of the diaphragm that drives the air out with forced expiration. Sometimes this seemingly automatic process doesn't function seamlessly. Most people today are shallow breathers, rarely thinking to strengthen, stretch, or train the diaphragm. It's automatic, right? Not really!

DIAGNOSES THAT CAN AFFECT THE DIAPHRAGM

The importance of the diaphragm's function is further revealed by the diagnoses that affect the diaphragm. For example, two-thirds of diagnoses of diaphragmatic paralysis are idiopathic (meaning with no known cause). An interruption of the diaphragm's nerve supply is one reported common cause. The nerve supply can be interrupted on one or both sides of the diaphragm; this can occur with lesions to the phrenic nerve, cervical spinal cord, or the brainstem. Other causes of diaphragmatic paralysis include surgery, accidents, cancerous or non-cancerous tumors, myopathies (myasthenia gravis), and neuropathies (diabetes).[10] Neck trauma and chiropractic manipulations could also be potential causes.[10] Many of these issues could arguably be fascial restrictions.

There are different degrees of diaphragmatic paralysis, just as with strokes or other nerve damage. Interestingly, paralysis of the affected side produces paradoxical movements of the abdominals. During paradoxical breathing, the diaphragm moves up with inhalation and down with exhalation, opposite of a normally functioning diaphragm.[10] Checking for paradoxical breathing is a way to test for healthy functioning of the diaphragm and a way to diagnose paralysis of the diaphragm.[10] Paradoxical breathing can also be seen in "healthy" individuals with poor breathing patterns. Clinically, I have seen paradoxically breathing following breast implants, heart surgeries, abdominal surgeries, and lobectomies, as well as in patients with poor posture and also in young and "healthy" athletes. Often we are able to reverse paradoxical breathing with education, exercises, and bodywork.

Another way to assess the quality and strength of the diaphragm is the sniff test.[10] A sniff is actually reflexive. When you sniff, the diaphragm should automatically move quickly outward and downward towards the pelvis. Someone with paralysis or a poor functioning diaphragm might not have this automatic response.

We can strengthen the diaphragm in the same way. Use your natural reflexes — sniff! This is good way to reflexively strengthen a weak diaphragm and to identify it with the "mind's eye" so to say. As we have discussed, these deep core muscles are hard to see and not always easy to activate and strengthen when weak.

Strengthening any of the deep core muscles would be beneficial for a person with a paralyzed diaphragm. Strengthening these muscles would also assist any athlete for optimal performance in their sport, especially if the diaphragm is their unidentified weak link, or maybe identified, but not given the proper attention. Are you looking to see if your diaphragm is at its full capacity?

Another way to test and analyze the diaphragm's function is via diagnostic ultrasound, looking for thickening of the diaphragm with inhalation.[11,12] This is another way to "see" the muscle.

The diaphragm is a critical muscle for staying alive. Nerve innervation for the diaphragm is from nerve roots at C3, C4, and C5 of the cervical spine.[13] As they say in anatomy class, "Three, four, five keep you alive." You never know when your system might need a little more life in it! Know where these deep core muscles are, know if they are *turned on,* and know how to turn them back on and/or enhance them. This can be life changing!

Just like all the other deep core muscles, the diaphragm is a stabilizer. Because the diaphragm separates the thoracic and abdominal contents, it allows pressure regulation between the two areas. Remember, *pressure* can provide *stability*. The diaphragm has the ability to provide stability when needed by controlling this pressure gradient. For example, the diaphragm muscle can provide an isometric contraction; contracting and holding the diaphragm muscle in one position limits pressure exchanges. This pressure holding allows stability, like the strength of an unopened soda pop can. Humans are better than a can; we are dynamic and can adjust our pressure/stability system. The diaphragm is in an optimal position to do this. One can see how the amount of lengthening and shortening of the muscle can indirectly manipulate the stability. The speed of the contraction can also manipulate the stability. For example, if you slowly exhale you can provide stability for a longer period of time, if needed. This will allow the core to both withstand more external pressure and provide more internal core stability.

Think about the importance of stability when a person is pushed. When someone is pushed, the diaphragm and other deep core muscles co-contract to provide stability for the body to resist the external force of the push. This example also shows how the deep core can provide stability for the legs. By helping the legs to ground the body to the earth, the deep core further stabilizes the body and prevents falling.

THE BODY CHOOSES TO BREATHE:
BREATH AND STABILITY

Hodges is well known in the field of physical therapy for his research linking the deep core, including the diaphragm, to stability.[14-16] One of his studies showed that when respiratory demands increase, the postural demands of the diaphragm decrease.[15] This makes sense — the body will choose to breathe to live! In physical therapy we use this knowledge to make changes in skeletal, muscular, and fascial systems. It can be quite amazing!

Let me share an amazing example. I don't have a video for this clinical experience, unfortunately. I'll try my best to describe it, but ultimately seeing was believing. Two years prior to coming to therapy, the patient had experienced an injury. Her lower intercostal muscles and diaphragm were dysfunctional, weak, and tight at the specific location of her original injury. The goal was to help the patient mobilize her lower intercostal muscles and diaphragm. We decided to maximize the potential of "the body will choose to breath" by isolating the diaphragm for breathing and recruiting all of the other deep core muscles to *stabilize*.

We asked the patient to use all of her breathing muscles *except* her diaphragm to stabilize herself so she wouldn't fall. When the breathing muscles are needed to stabilize, they will not be used to breathe. So she *had* to use her diaphragm that she had been guarding in order to breathe. In that moment, and the moments following, her ribs unraveled, her hips de-rotated (from internal rotation to external rotation), and her shoulders and body endured potentially hundreds of contractions. Twitching was going on everywhere. We were as shocked as the patient was. It was like a firework show of twitches. She stopped when she was ready. The whole event appeared extremely taxing and painful. But the results were amazing; she grew inches in seconds because of the trigger point and fascia releases. There were potentially hundreds of trigger point and myofascial releases. Unfortunately, this did leave her with a localized pain at her original injury in her lower ribs. However, we localized the pain, and she was on her way to healing more locally and with significantly less compensations.

THE DIAPHRAGM AS A STABLE PLATFORM

The diaphragm can act as a stable platform when the pelvis and lower back become weakened. In a healthy subject, many practitioners, including myself, will argue that the pelvis is the stable platform. However, what happens when it fails us? The diaphragm can act as a stable platform for a weak lumbopelvic junction. This is commonly seen in pregnant women who have less pelvic floor and lumbopelvic stability. The diaphragm will become a stabilizer for the legs to push and pull from and for the upper body to rest on. However, this is not an ideal situation!

THE DIAPHRAGM AND PREGNANCY

During pregnancy, the diaphragm is asked to do more! It is common to have decreased lumbopelvic stability during pregnancy. Excessive lumbar lordosis is a common posturing seen with pregnancy. Low back pain is also frequently experienced during pregnancy.

This lordotic positioning during pregnancy may further stretch the transverse abdominis muscle. Studies have shown that the rectus abdominis indeed does thin and elongate during pregnancy, and this is also what I see clinically.[17] Think of the excessive lordosis of the lumbar spine like reigns on a horse pulling to the front side of the body (the stomach). The reigns are the back muscles bending the vertebrae and stretching the stomach tissue. In this excessive lordotic position, the deep core is no longer in spine neutral. Again, remember, the deep core fires best when it is aligned. Furthermore, the pelvic floor has to withstand more pressure from baby, again weakening the maximal potential of the pelvic floor to assist with lumbopelvic stability. All of the above clinical findings tend to weaken the stability of the pelvis. When the lumbopelvic junction becomes unstable, the diaphragm may be asked to do more, specifically to do more stabilizing to make up for the weakened structures below. With more stabilizing, the diaphragm can become locked in a shortened or lengthened position, now affecting normal breathing. It is important to work on both minimizing and treating these common findings.

DIAPHRAGM AND CONTINENCE

Restoring the function of the diaphragm is another major area of assessment and treatment for many after delivery. What I have found clinically is that the diaphragm can sometimes be the leading culprit of incontinence. Why? The diaphragm becomes dysfunctional. Often it is shortened and/or functioning to stabilize the body instead of working to breathe. The position of the baby really does limit full expansion, especially at later trimesters, so it is not shocking that the diaphragm tends to function in a limited range of motion. The diaphragm, and really some of the lower intercostal muscles too, are no longer expanding to full lengths. The pressure system is in disarray. Where does all the pressure go with lifting, sneezing, and coughing when the diaphragm and lower intercostals are not fully expanding? The pressure goes down! Down to the lower abdominals, which are weakened, and to the pelvic floor. If you sneeze or cough, pay attention; your lower ribs and diaphragm should expand and the pelvic floor and the transverse abdominis should activate.

Lack of expansion at the diaphragm is a common abnormality seen in both pre- and postpartum parents even decades later. The muscle becomes less mobile and dynamic. Now the recoil/coil effect of the diaphragm is at stake. As a pelvic floor therapist, I commonly notice a lack of expansion at the lower intercostal muscles and the diaphragm with sneezing, coughing, laughing, and deep breathing. When these patients cough, for example, their lungs and upper abdominals are not expanding laterally, posteriorly, or anteriorly in a three hundred and sixty degree radius. Instead their very lower abdominals expand just above the pubic bone and they often report bladder leakage.

When the lower intercostal muscles and the diaphragm have become dysfunctional for whatever reason, the force from a sneeze, cough, jump, or run can go straight to the lower abdominal cavity. This pressure can also go to the pelvic floor, compressing the bladder and uterus, and leading to the leaking of urine or gas, and/or prolapse or increased risk of prolapse. Working on the dynamics and mobility of the diaphragm becomes an important part of therapy for treatment of urgency, urine stress incontinence, and prolapse.

VOIDING OF BOWEL MOVEMENTS AND URINE

The diaphragm offers assistance with gut motility, micturition of urine, and the voiding of bowel movements. As discussed previously, the diaphragm has ligamentous connections to the colon and intestines. One of the ways the diaphragm assists with gut motility is by moving the abdominal contents with exhalation/relaxation and inhalation/contraction. The diaphragm is constantly increasing and decreasing pressure on the abdominal contents, and this rhythmic change in pressure can help move food through the intestines and colon. This same movement can also act as a massage to the internal organs of the abdomen such as stomach, intestines, liver, and kidneys.

The isometric contraction of the diaphragm through its most downward or flattened position further assists with evacuation of bowel movements and/or urine. This position moves pressure downward towards the urethra and rectum to evacuate urine and bowel, respectively. In these ways, the diaphragm has the ability to assist in the prevention and treatment of constipation and the evacuation of the bowel.

PREVENTING CONSTIPATION, GERD,
AND MYOCARDIAL INFARCTION

Increased pressure in the abdominals has a direct relationship with increased pressure to both the esophagus and heart. This increased pressure correlates with both GERD and myocardial infarction (heart attacks) and can be caused by constipation. Preventing constipation through diaphragmatic breathing may help in prevention of GERD and myocardial infarction.

THE DIAPHRAGM AS A
GASTROINTESTINAL SPHINCTER

The crural diaphragm has been hypothesized to function biomechanically as a gastrointestinal sphincter to hold stomach content from entering the esophagus.[4] One of the two openings in the crural diaphragm is the esophageal hiatus. A hiatus is a hole or opening. The esophageal hiatus connects the esophagus to the stomach. The crural diaphragm muscle is believed to contract and assist with closing this hole to prevent stomach contents from going back up into the esophagus, causing stomach acid reflux or GERD.[4]

In one study, removal of the crural diaphragm in cats increased the frequency of spontaneous acid reflux.[5] This would indicate that the diaphragm has something to do with the prevention of stomach acid entering the esophagus. Clinically, when patients' diaphragms function well and mobility is restored, GERD symptoms reduce and/or subside.

THE DIAPHRAGM AND SWALLOWING

The crural diaphragm also assists with the swallowing of food. These muscle fibers have been shown to relax during swallowing.[4] The ability for the crural diaphragm muscle to relax makes it easier for food to enter the stomach. Interestingly, studies are showing that the crural diaphragm acts as a doorkeeper, opening and closing with the body's demands.[4]

PREVENTION OF ESOPHAGEAL HERNIA

The contraction of the diaphragm during inspiration assists to close the stomach at the lower esophageal sphincter. This prevents the stomach from expelling food into the esophagus, creating stomach acid reflux and pain, and eventually deterioration of the esophageal lining and/or development of a hernia. When the diaphragm contracts, it moves away from the lung cavity and takes pressure off of the esophagus. It is important that the diaphragm is not stuck up in the lungs, immobile and pushing on the esophagus.

With an esophageal hernia, the stomach goes past the diaphragm and lower esophageal sphincter and into the esophagus. The door is broken. In order to assist in the prevention of a hernia, it is important to have a strong and *mobile* diaphragm and deep core.

THE DIAPHRAGM AND CIRCULATION

The esophagus is not the only structure that runs through the crural diaphragm. The aorta also does so. This is the biggest artery, supplying oxygenated blood to the pelvis and legs. The aorta is positioned nice and deep, in front of the spine, and goes directly through the diaphragm between the two crural legs. Because of the aorta's positioning, the high pressure area of the diaphragm minimally affects it. Therefore, it is able to passively supply blood to the low pressure areas of the legs.

The inferior vena cava, a large vein that takes deoxygenated blood back to the heart, passes through the top of the dome of the diaphragm and through the tendinous portion of the muscle. Thus, the inferior vena cava is not squeezed by the bulk of the diaphragm muscle. With inhalation, the diaphragm goes down into the stomach, abdominal pressure increases, thoracic pressure decreases, and the inferior vena cava can now act like a straw, drawing up deoxygenated blood from the legs. In this way, the diaphragm aids in the body's circulation.

THE NATURAL DECOMPRESSION SYSTEM

The diaphragm is another part of the deep core constantly providing decompression for the spine and vertebrae. As discussed in previous chapters, with every inhalation, the vertebrae and discs have the potential to be decompressed.

ANXIETY

Clinically, patients diagnosed with anxiety often report that they feel they cannot take a full breath. With therapy, hands-on skills, and exercises, the patient and I are able to restore normal breathing function and decrease and/or eliminate anxiety. Often they will say, "I told the doctor I couldn't breathe and if I could I wouldn't have anxiety." I believe patients with anxiety diagnoses should be assessed for muscular and fascial restrictions for the CAUSE and CURE of their anxiety.

THE IMPORTANCE OF FULL DIAPHRAGMATIC MOBILITY

Just as with all the other deep core muscles, it is important to keep full mobility of the diaphragm. Remember, anything restricting the diaphragm from moving down, up, out, or in *will* restrict its full ability to contract. It *will* restrict your full potential to breathe and stabilize and all the other functions of the diaphragm. Elements that commonly restrict downward motion of the diaphragm are our own internal forces, such as the abdominal muscles being held in a contracted and shortened state, which will stop the diaphragm from moving freely. Unfortunately, many people think and are fooled by the illusion of a tight core equaling a strong core. Even highly educated physical therapists are fooled by this falsehood. TIGHT DOES NOT MEAN STRONG, DYNAMIC, AND FUNCTIONAL. In fact, it can mean the exact opposite. It is attractive to have a tight stomach until it is not, because first and foremost you need to have mobility! If you are always holding the abdominal muscles, they are not working to their full capacity. In time, they will become dysfunctional and alter the function of surrounding tissues. An inflamed or obese gut is another diaphragm restriction. In a different manner, a weak gut (muscularly or fascially) will not allow full expansion with inhalation and/or fully assisted exhalation.

THE DANCE OF THE DEEP CORE

When you breathe in, the diaphragm moves down, the abdominal muscles, including the transverse abdominis, lengthen, and the pelvic floor also lengthens. The intercostal muscles, if they are pliable, allow lateral and anterior/posterior expansion of the diaphragm. The multifidi allow space to open between the discs and vertebrae of the spine and, indirectly, allow space to open between the ribs. Can you see how the deep core is dancing together?

THE DIAPHRAGM INTERACTS
WITH OTHER MUSCLES

Muscles that commonly affect the normal mobility of the diaphragm are the quadratus lumborum, intercostals, multifidi, long muscles of the spine (erector spinae), latissimus dorsi, and the abdominal muscles.

The long muscles of the spine can restrict posterior expansion of the diaphragm. If the latissimus dorsi muscle or the erector spinae muscles are tight, the diaphragm will have to fight their resistance. The truth is that many times the diaphragm will not fight; it will take the path of least resistance. Even the multifidi and, indirectly, the ability of the vertebral joints to be mobile, will affect the diaphragm, specifically at L1–L2 where the crural ligaments of the diaphragm connect to the vertebrae.

It is not uncommon clinically to see patients who are locked up in the back due to a direct fall who develop asthma immediately or shortly after their injury (within a year). Furthermore, GERD can also be associated with lack of mobility at the vertebrae. Remember that the crural tendons of the diaphragm attach at this level.

USE YOUR DIAPHRAGM TO
FIGHT YOUR INTERNAL RESTRICTIONS

You CAN force the diaphragm to fight through tight tissues. You can do this with exercises and with thought. Mentally and physically, you can cause the diaphragm and the surrounding tissues to lengthen and shorten. You can use your breath to mobilize your ribs and push past your restrictive internal forces. The diaphragm muscle can provide the strength and space for things to move, stretch, and realign; therefore it is important to keep it mobile and strong.

THE DIAPHRAGM AND LOW BACK PAIN

Abnormal diaphragm position is correlated with low back pain.[18] A study by Kolar et al. demonstrated that decreased diaphragmatic excursion is correlated with increased low back pain.[18] And a study by Janssens et al. showed greater diaphragmatic fatiguability in individuals with low back pain.[19] All of the deep core muscles, including the diaphragm, work together to both stabilize your body and to breathe, assisting in alignment and in decompression of the spine. It is therefore not surprising that problems with the diaphragm are associated with low back pain.

HOW DO YOU KNOW IF THE DIAPHRAGM IS *TURNED ON?*

Look and Feel Closely

Assess to see if the diaphragm is turned on by looking at your lower ribs and upper abdominals. Simply look to see if they are moving outward on all sides of your body. Do you feel the diaphragm go down in your rib cage with inhalation and upward with exhalation?

Sniff Test

It's time to run some tests on you. Start with the reflex test, the sniff test. Sniff and then feel for a normal response. A normal response would be the diaphragm quickly moving downward towards your pelvis. This would be felt below your sternum and at the border of your ribs on the front side.

Circumferential Measurement

For the next test you can lie down, sit, or stand. Place your hand on your upper abdominal muscles. When you inhale, does your circumference expand outward on all sides of your body at your lower ribs, just below your sternum, and also at your belly, halfway between your sternum and umbilicus? When lying down on your back, you should feel your upper abdominals move upwards to the sky, downwards to your feet, and outward to your sides and your back. Remember, a weak or paralyzed diaphragm might cause paradoxical breathing, where the lower ribs and upper abdomen move inward upon inhalation. This would be a sign that the diaphragm is not *turned on*.

You can also measure this movement. With a flexible tape measure, measure the difference in your circumference between full exhalation and full inhalation. Take the circumferential measurement halfway between the xiphoid process and the umbilicus (see chapter "Intercostals"). Your circumference should increase with inhalation.

Vocal Command

In general, for a long inhale and exhale movement of the diaphragm, you want to think light and long, gentle and quiet. However, when identifying and assessing if the muscle is *turned on*, quick movements are often more noticeable. With a quick vocal command, say "ah!" out loud and feel for a quick contraction of your diaphragm. Quickly say "ah!". You should feel the diaphragm move down and reflexively back up. Then say "ah!" loudly followed by "sss". With the "sss" you should feel the recoil of the diaphragm going back up into the ribs. The ability to feel these movements is a sign that the diaphragm is *turned on*.

The diaphragm also has the power to turn others on! The diaphragm is a vocal muscle and a strong voice is attractive. The diaphragm also has the ability to ignite life in the deep core and to promote attractive, lively, and youthful movements.

HOW CAN YOU *TURN ON* THE DIAPHRAGM?

Focus on Feeling

When doing these exercises, focus on feeling kinesthetically and with your hands. With a slow inhalation, feel for the diaphragm to move down in your ribs and out on all sides of your body. Feel for your lower ribs to expand, feel for your upper abdominal and mid back muscles lengthen. With the exhale, focus on the upper abdominal muscles and skin drawing back in, the ribs coming to midline, and the diaphragm going back into a domed position in the ribs. When getting started, try to be in a relaxed place and state of mind. Think light, soft, and gentle.

Sniff Reflex

As with the lower intercostal muscles, you can use sniffs to assist in activating the diaphragm. Start with a short sniff, then wait five seconds while relaxing. Feel for the diaphragm to recoil back into the ribs during those five seconds. Repeat ten times. Progress to a five-second sniff with a five- to ten-second rest in between. Progress your sniffs over days, weeks, months, or years to ten seconds. The inhale part of the sniffs should become easy, slow, and effortless with consistent outward expansion of the diaphragm.

Another way to use sniffing for strengthening the diaphragm is to do one short sniff, one longer sniff, and one longest sniff; do all sniffs without exhaling. Then exhale and rest before repeating again. Progress to repetitions of ten and do six sets a day for lasting results. Mass practice is necessary for neurological and muscular changes, as mentioned in previous chapters.

Tummy Movement

Place a toy on your upper tummy, below your sternum, and move it with your diaphragm as you breathe. This is a classical way to improve diaphragmatic breathing. If you don't want to play with a toy, just imagine that you are moving an object on your tummy with your diaphragm.

Make It a Lifestyle

Focus on inhaling slowly and deeply throughout the day. Try to draw in as much air as you can and then slowly exhale as much air as you can. Try to use less and less effort, quieting it, but yet getting to end ranges with both inhalation and exhalation.

Position for Success

Placing yourself in a flexed position will assist in activating the diaphragm. Child's pose, bent over in fetal position with buttocks on your heels, is an example. I like to use this position to focus on the posterior/back expansion of the diaphragm. Or, while lying on your side in bed, bend inward at the spine. Just sitting and placing your head down and bending forward is an easy position in which to focus on the diaphragm. Riding on a stationary bike with your head down and upper back flexed is another more active position. Gazing down assists with the diaphragm posteriorly expanding. Hand placement can help too.

Strength Progression of the Diaphragm

Some progressions have already been discussed, such as holding sniffs longer with inhalation or doing more sniffs with one inhalation. Another progression already discussed is coming to end range inhalation and exhalation and getting there slower and with less effort. Just as with the intercostal muscles, strengthening could involve holding end range efforts, or holding midrange efforts for isometric strengthening.

Inhaling for x amount of time and then exhaling for more than that amount, and vice versa, is another way to progress. Holding inhalation for less time and exhalation for more time will focus on end range exhalation, the eccentric movement of the diaphragm. More inhalation time than exhalation time will improve concentric strength of the diaphragm and end range inhalation. Remember, with end ranges we can also work to stretch not only the diaphragm muscle itself, but also the surrounding fascia and muscles.

Adding resistance is another way to make the diaphragm work harder. You could do this with a resistance band or with your hands. You could wrap a resistance band around the diaphragm, below the sternum, and try to expand out into it. Attempt to stretch the band with your diaphragm. Weightlifting in and of itself is another way to strengthen this stabilizing muscle. Stabilization and balance exercises can also assist to strengthen the diaphragm.

Use the Diaphragm to Turn On the Pelvic Floor Muscles

The diaphragm can be used to turn your pelvic floor on! It can assist in elongation and lengthening of the pelvic floor (see chapter "Pelvic Floor"). This elongation can be used to assist in releasing tight pelvic floor muscles. Furthermore, the diaphragmatic contraction can be used reflexively to restore the dynamics of the pelvic floor. Remember, the diaphragmatic motion and contraction of the pelvic floor muscles function together for normal breathing.

REFERENCES

1. Bordoni B, Zanier E. Anatomical connections of the diaphragm: Influence of respiration on the body system. *Journal of Multidisciplinary Healthcare.* 2013;6:281-91. doi:10.2147/jmdh.s45443

2. Kolar P, Neuwirth J, Sanda J, et al. Analysis of diaphragm movement during tidal breathing and during its activation while breath holding using MRI synchronized with spirometry. *Physiological Research.* 2009;58:383-92. doi:10.33549/physiolres.931376

3. Kolar P, Sulc J, Kyncl M, et al. Stabilizing function of the diaphragm: Dynamic MRI and synchronized spirometric

assessment. *Journal of Applied Physiology.* 2010;109: 1064-71. doi:10.1152/japplphysiol.01216.2009

4. Mittal RK. The crural diaphragm, an external lower esophageal sphincter: A definitive study. *Gastroenterology.* 1993;105:1565-7. doi:10.1016/0016-5058(93)90167-b

5. Mittal RK, Sivri B, Schirmer BD, Heine KJ. Effect of crural myotomy on the incidence and mechanism of gastroesophageal reflux in cats. *Gastroenterology.* 1993;105:740-7. doi:10.1016/0016-5085(93)90891-f

6. Pickering M, Jones JFX. The diaphragm: Two physiological muscles in one. *Journal of Anatomy.* 2002;201:305-12. doi:10.1046/j.1469-7580.2002.00095.x

7. Gorman N. Diaphragm. Kenhub. September 19, 2023. Accessed May 20, 2025. www.kenhub.com/en/library/anatomy/diaphragm

8. Gray H. *Anatomy of the Human Body.* 20th ed. Lewis WH, ed. Lea & Febiger; 1918. Accessed May 20, 2025. https://archive.org/details/anatomyofhumanbo1918gray/mode/2up

9. Nassar S, Menias CO, Palmquist S, et al. Ligament of Treitz: Anatomy, relevance of radiologic findings, and radiologic-pathologic correlation. *American Journal of Roentgenology.* 2021;216:927-934. doi:10.2214/AJR.20.23273

10. Ben-Dov I. Diaphragmatic paralysis — symptoms, evaluation, therapy and outcome. In: Molloy E, ed. *Congenital Diaphragmatic Hernia: Prenatal to Childhood Management and Outcomes.* IntechOpen; 2012. Accessed May 20, 2025. https://www.intechopen.com/chapters/37827.

11. Goligher EC, Laghi F, Detsky ME, et al. Measuring diaphragm thickness with ultrasound in mechanically ventilated patients: feasibility, reproducibility and validity. *Intensive Care Medicine.* 2015;41:642-9. doi:10.1007/s00134-015-3687-3

12. Carrillo-Esper R, Pérez-Calatayud ÁA, Arch-Tirado E, et al. Standardization of sonographic diaphragm thickness evaluations in healthy volunteers. *Respiratory Care.* 2016;61:920-4. doi:10.4187/respcare.03999

13. Merrell AJ, Kardon G. Development of the diaphragm — a skeletal muscle essential for mammalian respiration. *FEBS Journal.* 2013;280:4026-35. doi:10.1111/febs.12274

14. Hodges PW, Gandevia SC. Changes in intra-abdominal pressure during postural and respiratory activation of the human diaphragm. *Journal of Applied Physiology.* 2000;89:967–76. doi:10.1152/jappl.2000.89.3.967

15. Hodges PW, Heijnen I, Gandevia SC. Postural activity of the diaphragm is reduced in humans when respiratory demand increases. *Journal of Physiology.* 2001;537:999–1008. doi:10.1111/j.1469-7793.2001.00999.x

16. Hodges PW, Sapsford R, Pengel LHM. Postural and respiratory functions of the pelvic floor muscles. *Neurourology and Urodynamics.* 2007;26:362-71. doi:10.1002/nau.20232

17. Coldron Y, Stokes MJ, Newham DJ, Cook K. Postpartum characteristics of rectus abdominis on ultrasound imaging. *Manual Therapy.* 2008;13:112-21. doi:10.1016/j.math.2006.10.001

18. Kolar P, Sulc J, Kyncl M, et al. Postural function of the

diaphragm in persons with and without chronic low back pain. *Journal of Orthopaedic and Sports Physical Therapy.* 2012;42,4: 352-62. doi:10.2519/jospt.2012.3830

19. Janssens L, Brumagne S, McConnel AK, et al. Greater diaphragm fatigability in individuals with recurrent low back pain. *Respiratory Physiology & Neurobiology.* 2013;188:119-23. doi:10.1016/j.resp.2013.05.028

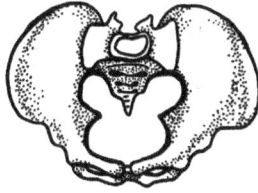

VOCAL CORDS

The vocal cords, also known as the vocal folds, are located in your throat within the larynx at the top of the trachea (Figure 7.1). The vocal cords are protected behind your Adam's apple or thyroid cartilage at cervical vertebral levels three through five. They run horizontally from back to front across the larynx. The vocal cords open and close; in anatomical terms, they respectively abduct and adduct. There are a multitude of small muscles and structures that help control this opening and closing.

The "true" vocal cords are a pair of two bands that stretch horizontally across the larynx. They are fibrous and tough in nature. The "false" vocal cords are also known as the ventricular folds. They are two thick folds of mucus membrane (see Figure 7.2).[1] The false vocal cords are located within the larynx, superior to the true vocal cords.

Interestingly, the vocal cords are sixty percent smaller in females than in males. This is a higher percentage than for any other body part in comparison.[2] This size difference assists with our ability to identify female and male voices.

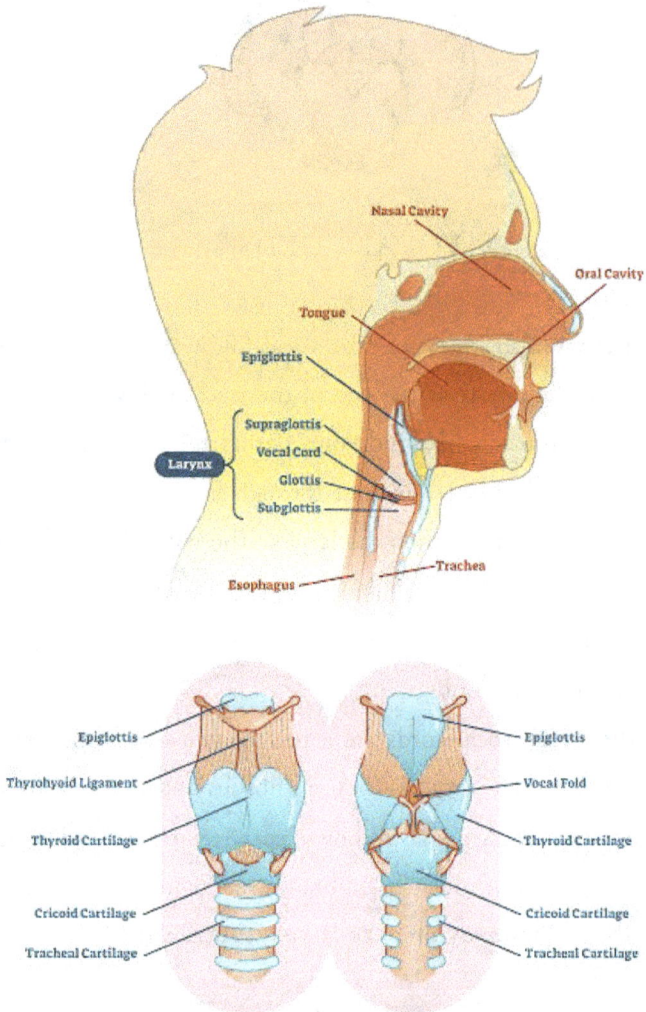

Figure 7.1. The larynx.
Adapted from VectorMine/*Shutterstock.com.*

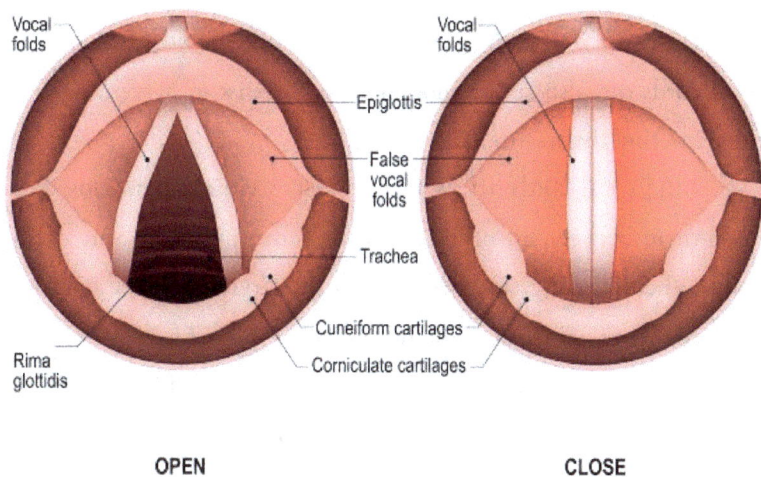

Figure 7.2. The vocal cords are also called the vocal folds.
From Disignua/*Shutterstock.com*.

VOCAL CORDS ARE PART OF OUR AIRWAY PATH

When you breathe, air enters through either the nose or the mouth. Then air goes into the pharynx, which is like a common space or junction where the nose, mouth, and larynx openings come together. There are two pathways at the pharynx for anything entering the mouth or nose to travel through: the digestive pathway (via the esophagus) or the airway (through the larynx and into the trachea). When you say "my food went down the wrong tube," you are implying that your food entered the trachea and not the esophagus; this is when choking or coughing can occur.

When food is swallowed, the food pushes the epiglottis (a flap in the larynx) backward (see Figure 7.3). The epiglottis acts as a door, closing the opening of the trachea (windpipe). The epiglottis has connections to your tongue, hyoid bone, and thyroid cartilage. The vocal cords can also act as another door to assist in preventing food from entering the trachea.

The vocal cords act as a *valve* that is either open, closed, or somewhere between in order to let air move in and/or out of the body. When inhaling, air goes through the larynx, past the open vocal cords to the trachea, and then into the bronchioles within the lungs. The vocal cords can trap air inside and/or outside the body by closing. This is one mechanical way that *stability* is created for our core.

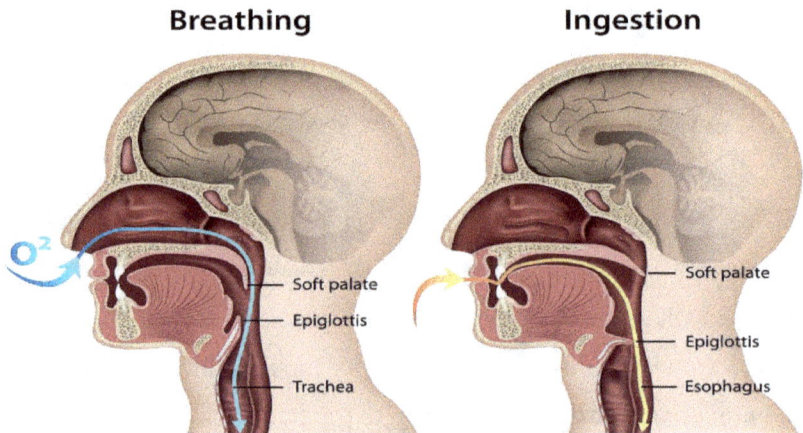

Figure 7.3. The epiglottis acts as a door.
From Medicalstocks/*Shutterstock.com.*

WHAT ARE VOCAL CORDS?

The vocal cords consist of many layers. The first layer is the squamous epithelium. Below this layer is subepithelial connective tissue and the vocal ligament. The vocalis and thyroarytenoid muscles make up the deepest layer.[3,4] The vocalis muscle is the main muscle of the vocal cords and it runs parallel with the vocal ligament (see Figure 7.4). The vocal cords form the opening of the throat called the rima glottidis.[1]

The muscles at the larynx can be divided into extrinsic and intrinsic muscles.[1] The intrinsic laryngeal muscles alter both *the length and the tension* and *the opening and closing* of the vocal cords. The intrinsic muscles include the posterior and lateral cricoarytenoid muscles, arytenoid muscles, cricothyroid muscle, and the thyroarytenoid muscles. The posterior cricoarytenoid muscles abduct, pulling the vocal cords away from midline and therefore *opening the airway.* The lateral cricoarytenoid and arytenoid muscles *close the vocal cords.*[1,5,6]

The extrinsic laryngeal muscles assist to *support* the larynx within the cervical region; they *move the larynx* as a whole.[5] The extrinsic muscles include the digastric muscle, stylohyoid muscle, mylohyoid muscle, geniohyoid muscle, hyoglossus muscle, and genioglossus muscle, sternohyoid muscle, sternothyroid muscle, thyrohyoid muscle, and omohyoid muscle.[6]

Combining all of the intrinsic and extrinsic laryngeal muscles, you can see that there are a lot of muscles that assist with the opening and closing of the airway. But the actual doors could be viewed as the vocal cords. Nevertheless, when we speak of vocal cord function, it is really all of these laryngeal muscles that assist in *controlling* the doors. All parts are working together, some just get more credit as they are at the forefront!

Origin: Lateral surface of the vocal processes of the arytenoid cartilage.

Insertion: Anterior part of the vocal ligament (ipsilaterally, on the same side).

Action: Tenses anterior part and relaxes posterior part of the vocal ligament.[4]

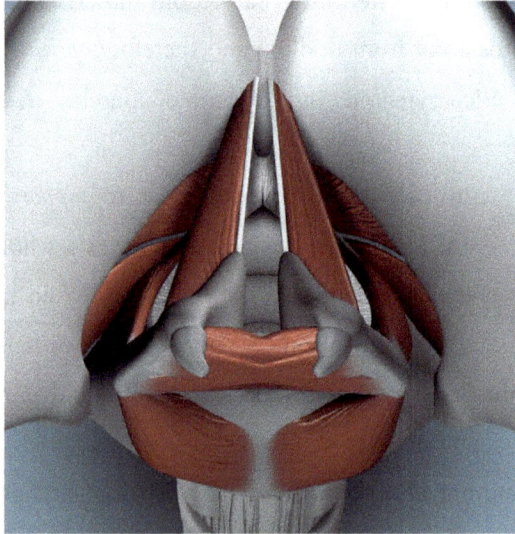

Figure 7.4. The vocalis muscle.
From Yifeng Xuan/*Shutterstock.com.*

WHY ARE THE VOCAL CORDS SO IMPORTANT?

The vocal cords have six main functions. They assist with vocalization. They assist with breathing. They also assist with stability, postural control, and evacuation of bowel and bladder due to their ability to trap air in the thoracic cavity. And the vocal cords assist in the prevention of choking.

The vocal cords are the opening and closing of your airway into your lungs. The larynx acts as a pressure valve that is *so powerful,* with the vocal cords being the more direct anatomical means to open and/or close the connection between the outside and inside of your body.

BREATHING AND VOCAL CORD DYSFUNCTION

Sometimes the best way to understand the importance of a muscle, as any system, is to look at a dysfunctional system. Vocal cord dysfunction is a condition in which the vocal cords are not moving the way they should. This is also known as paradoxical vocal cord dysfunction. Just as with the pelvic floor, the diaphragm, and the intercostal muscles, the vocal cords have the potential to become paradoxical, in that they are moving opposite the direction they should be *with breathing.*

Normally, the vocal cords should open to allow air to come in with inhalation and they should come closer together with exhalation. With paradoxical breathing, this is reversed.

Symptoms of vocal cord dysfunction can be a tight throat, tight chest, and a vibrating sensation in the throat. Sounds that can be heard are whizzing, striding, and even sounds of choking. Obviously when you cannot breathe signs of anxiety might also be displayed. Other symptoms that have been reported and seen are chest tightness, pain, and feelings of lightheadedness. Not being able to get a deep enough breath in and/or feelings of not having the endurance of other similarly trained athletes are other potential symptoms of vocal cord dysfunction.

No clear pathology for vocal cord dysfunction has been identified, *so they say*. Vocal cord dysfunction is often misdiagnosed as asthma as the symptoms are similar; however, the same treatment often does not work. It is important to treat the cause, not just the symptoms! If you really think about it, most medical diagnoses are just bodily symptoms and signs.

My theory with vocal cord dysfunction is that one of the causes is poor myofascial and skeletal alignment and mobility. The throat is just fascia, more tissue. The tissue (bone, cartilage, collagen, muscles, arteries, nerves) becomes misaligned, tight, taut. Just like a tight hamstring, the tissue might start to pull and/or spasm, or change normal biomechanics. When you go to breathe in, the tissue might restrict instead of opening, just like the hamstring might contract or spasm when attempting to lengthen. The throat has much more detrimental consequences — no oxygen.

A PERSONAL STORY

Why might problems be going on in the vocal cords? How does one develop myofascial and skeletal alignment issues? This answer will vary for each individual. For example, my son was born with tongue-tie. On top of having tongue-tie, he also had his tonsils and adenoids removed. He was exposed to the trauma of surgery at a muscle and fascial level related to his vocal cords.

Spiritually, it is possible that my son comes from a past life of not speaking up for things he wants and/or needs. I used to have to constantly ask him if he would like anything while my other son just tells me effortlessly. He still needs to be reminded to ask and to speak up. He is changing his behavior, as he knows that his past life does not need to affect his current lifetime. When someone is resisting something at a mental or spiritual level, many times this shows up at a physical level as well. For my son, this shows up in his throat and tongue.

Surgery in and of itself could be another cause of myofascial imbalances. After the surgery to remove his tonsils and adenoids, my son developed a clot that caused a small bit of blood. He went to the sink to spit and had less than a drop of blood. His group of doctors associated with Children's Hospital of Wisconsin did not do follow ups unless a parent or child reported blood. However, they appeared to live in fear that clots post tonsillectomy would bleed out. So, any bit of blood accompanying a clot led to another surgery, even though they really had no way of knowing how many kids with tonsillectomies actually had a clot nor how many actually bled. Nevertheless, when we reported blood, they said it was an emergency and they needed to prepare for another surgery. I had no time to determine if they were correct. I was left to trust the doctors. They took him into surgery again when he had still not recovered physically or at his surgical site from the first one.

The fourth day post second throat surgery, a little tiny drop of blood came out when my son spit after brushing his teeth. He cried. I took him to the hospital again but I refused that they do a third surgery. They agreed to keep him overnight, but said surgery would be necessary if he bled again. I had one night to research. I found dozens of pictures showing blood clots post operation days one through twelve and even up to day thirty. In these pictures, one could see patients' wounds and clots healing in their throats without surgery.

The next morning, I told the doctors that there were numerous people recovering from this surgery with clots without surgery. But the doctors described the worst, my son having this clot and then bleeding uncontrollably out into his airway. The doctors noted that he had a few drops of blood on his pillow and they insisted that we do a third surgery.

While my son was in surgery, I spoke with my brother-in-law who was working as a resident with an Ear, Nose, and Throat (ENT) doctor. ENT doctors do tonsillectomies. My brother-in-law said that they do follow ups and see a bit of blood now and then, but they don't do unnecessary surgeries. This makes logical sense.

My son had three surgeries, two without my true consent or understanding. I say true consent in that yes, I signed a piece of paper allowing the surgery to happen, but I was not willing.

The doctors said that they needed to do it. Honestly, I don't think they would have let me leave with my child if we wanted to. This was scary and still is scary! Unfortunately, many unnecessary surgeries take place, by choice and not by choice! We were not left with a choice! These surgeries led to increased recovery time and could have led to vocal cord dysfunction or scar tissue restrictions, most likely restricting the function of his laryngeal muscles. Additionally, the doctors gave me no clarity about what the follow-up surgeries entailed. What exactly did they do? They were not clear.

Again, you might ask why people have vocal cord dysfunction. Some people might be born with tight musculature, others might be restricting themselves due to prior experiences or trauma, and for others, maybe doctors did it to them. Anything that affects alignment and the myofascial system could interfere with the function of your vocal cords. Even viral and bacterial infections could affect the laryngeal muscles and limit the potential of the vocal cords.

BREATHING: THE VITAL JOB OF THE VOCAL CORDS

Vocal cord dysfunction, as mentioned previously, affects breathing. These individuals can struggle with asthma-like symptoms at rest or with activity/sport. The ability to let air both in and out can be affected. The laryngeal muscles are so crucial to vitality; they must be turned on and must be able to open and close. Just as with a muscle or fascia in your hamstrings or quadriceps, when the laryngeal muscles/fascia are tight or dysfunctional, they can lock up. Do you want this happening in your throat!? Let's keep the vocal cords and their associated muscles and fascia healthy. "Healthy" means free of restrictions and able to move to end ranges. Healthy also means the ability to have some strength and power behind movements. Most importantly, make sure these muscles are *turned on* to meet your body's demands!

Currently, clinics in the United States are starting to retrain the laryngeal muscles using biofeedback via imaging at the vocal cords. This imaging provides the ability to see the vocal cords in real time, meaning the vocal cords can be seen in motion while doing functional movements. Imaging can be used for therapeutic exercises and for diagnostic purposes. The patient is able to *see* their deep core muscles functioning. Unfortunately, imaging is minimally offered and it is also intrusive and expensive.

Imaging is just one part of fixing the problem. Seeing and diagnosing is one thing, but ultimately functional range of motion must be restored at the vocal cords and the laryngeal musculature. Some of this can be done with therapeutic, vocal cord, and laryngeal exercises, speech therapy, and vocal lessons. However, for more complete and effective treatment, I would also recommend correcting alignment at the vocal cords and also at the surrounding muscle and myofascial restrictions. When bone, muscle, and fascia are aligned, the deep core fires better! When aligned, the deep core is positioned for success.

It is common clinically to see muscle and fascial restrictions at the cervical spine and surrounding tissues with people who have difficulty with speech and difficulty swallowing. It is also common to see improvements in their speech and swallowing with corrections in the musculoskeletal limitations found in their neck. I have further noticed that correcting the alignment of the body overall and improving the function of the other deep core muscles also enhances the function of the vocal cords. I use bodywork (hands-on therapy) to correct alignment at the mouth, tongue, throat, chest, and thoracic region for vocal cord issues.

PERFORMANCE AND YOUR VOCAL CORDS

As mentioned in previous chapters, the soda pop can theory refers to the way that pressure can keep the body upright and stable, much like an unopened can of soda. The vocal cords act as a door. Closing them prevents air from entering or exiting, which allows for dynamic stability. This is also known as air trapping.[7] The vocal cords have been observed to almost consistently close with increased power demand in the upper extremities with vault and horizontal bar exercises.[8] Having the ability to close your vocal cords allows for *power, power beyond your throat.* The deep core offers power for stabilization within your core, which indirectly affects power to your extremities. Consider your neck as an extremity.

VOCAL CORDS AND PHONATION

Your vocal cords create harmonics, many pitches of sound in the form of waves of energy. Sound waves move through the air much like the ripples that occur when a drop of rain hits a still lake. The most common wave form that you produce is the pitch at which you are considered to be singing and/or speaking.

Sound is created by vibration traveling from the vocal cords in the throat and out of the mouth. The vocal cords themselves have the ability to vibrate at high frequencies visible to special high-speed photography, but not visible to the naked eye. This vibration is created by our breath.

The throat itself can take on a unique form (see Figure 7.5). Some of this form can be manipulated by surrounding tissues, which helps to dictate the sound that is heard. Genetics, of course, also plays a role in the form of the throat and therefore our phonation. Enhancing the mobility, strength, and alignment of the vocal cords and surrounding tissue assists in phonation. How one uses the deep core and the pressure system of the deep core will also have an effect on phonation.

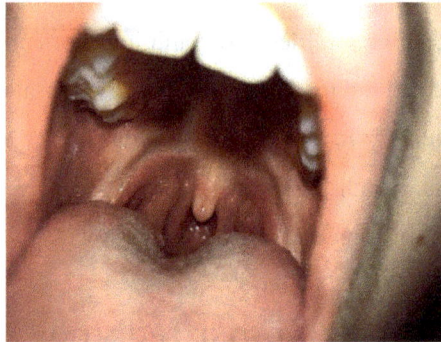

Figure 7.5. The throat.
From Another Average Joe/*Shutterstock.com.*

I have seen some interesting compensations for phonation. When one of my patients would say her name, I could see the long muscles of her spine contract like keys moving on a piano. This is still a mystery to me, but for some reason she was using her back muscles to talk, specifically the iliocostalis, longissimus, and spinalis muscles bilaterally. Why? Most likely her deep core muscles were not functioning to their full ability and were less capable of regulating pressure. Unfortunately, I did not get to study this patient for very long, as her reason for therapy was solved in a few visits. Many times I have more things I want to fix than a patient cares to even acknowledge.

WHO ELSE HAS PROBLEMS WITH THEIR VOCAL CORDS?

People are commonly referred to therapists in order to work on the muscles of the throat and tongue if they have difficulty swallowing food, a current or past history of choking, or difficulty speaking. People are referred to therapists less commonly, unfortunately, for breathing problems, enlarged tonsils or adenoids, pain in the throat, tongue-tie, and vocal cord dysfunction. Trauma to the throat and viral illnesses are other causes of weak vocal cords and potentially appropriate reasons for therapy.

Individuals who talk or sing a lot are also at risk of developing weak and dysfunctional vocal cords. Teachers, coaches, and public speakers are examples of people who can develop weak and inflamed vocal cords. If you think about it, inflamed vocal cords are like a tendonitis of the vocal cords and the associated muscles. Rest, cold and heat therapy, bodywork, exercises, and neuromuscular re-education are all applicable.

People whose voices are not strong or who are not sounding like their normal self should also consider seeing a therapist for improved vocal cord function. I had one male patient who was scheduled to have surgery secondary to a high, squeaky voice. I focused on eliminating muscle, fascial, and bony alignment restrictions in this patient's neck and throat. These therapies, combined with a referral to a speech therapist for voice exercises, provided significant improvement in this patient's ability to speak. He was happy to get his manly voice back and to return to public speaking. Voice is a big deal, as those compromised will be sure to inform you! How is your vocal image? Are you vocally attractive? Are you *turned on?* Can you turn on others with your vocal cords?

Singers are a group of people who are very interested in their vocal cords for optimization of phonation. They are true athletes, requiring speed, agility, coordination, flexibility, and endurance at the laryngeal muscles. Would strengthening these muscles be beneficial for any human or athlete, just like the rest of the deep core? There are not many studies or clinical practices known to me at this time that discuss strengthening the vocal cords and laryngeal muscles for improved quality of life or sport. However, maybe we should consider doing this.

VOCAL CORDS AND PNEUMONIA

Aspiration occurs when food gets past the vocal cords and enters the lungs. Regular aspiration is capable of causing pneumonia and infections due to foreign objects in the lungs. Less likely, a single case of aspiration could cause infections or pneumonia. It is clearly important that we are able to close the vocal cords, to come to full adduction, to prevent choking. Making sure that the vocal cords have full mobility is important, as with any deep core muscle.

First, find your thyroid cartilage. Place two fingers on the front of your neck at the top of your throat. Now swallow and you should feel a hard nodule move up. Yawn and you should feel that nodule move down. This is your thyroid cartilage. Your vocal cords are behind this cartilaginous tissue. You should be able to lightly move your thyroid cartilage from side to side.

Your vocal cords naturally activate when coughing or when clearing your throat. This should be reflexive. So violently clear your throat with the goal of discovering your vocal cords. Feel for them to close; you will not be able to breathe in at this time as the airway is closed. This is not an exercise, but rather a way to identify the vocal cords. Take note of the vocal cords coming together. Another way to feel the vocal cords come together is to stick out your tongue while clearing your throat.

The vocal cords abduct and adduct. Abduct means they move apart and adduct means they come together. Controlling the amount of abduction and adduction can alter your pressure system and phonation. Now try to identify the vocal cords opening! Make some noises! When you say "sss", the vocal cords should open and therefore abduct. When you say "zzz", the vocal cords vibrate. When you say "eee", the vocal cords come closer together and assist with phonation. You can better "see" and "feel" your vocal cords working by closing your eyes. You can also plug your ears.

Swelling at the vocal cords is a sign that your vocal cords are weakened or not *turned on*. Check to see if you have any swelling in your throat. Again, teachers, coaches, singers, and people overusing their voice are at a regular risk for developing inflammation and impaired function of their vocal cords, just like a runner is at risk of developing achilles or patella tendonitis or any inflammation at their overworked muscles, tendons, joints and/or fascia. Besides feeling and observing for swelling in the neck, you can assess via speech. Higher pitches than usual can be a sign of swelling. Inability to hold a vocal task that is very soft can also be a sign of swelling. With singing, you might notice squeakiness or an inability to reach high or low pitches. Inflammation is a sign of tissue damage and affects the ability of muscles to fire and function. These are signs that your vocal cords are not turned on!

Pain at the throat is another obvious sign that the vocal cords are not happy. It is common to have swelling in the throat when you are sick, and, if this is the case, it is important to let the throat fully heal. You do not want to let the inflammation become chronic. Ease back into using your voice. Do some vocal cord exercises. Just as with any other ligament, muscle, and/or tendon, take the load off and progress load and duration as you are able.

S/Z Ratio

The S/Z Ratio Test is a measure of the ability to open and close the vocal cords and the range of motion of the vocal cords. Making an "sss" sound uses the open, or abducted position of the vocal cords. Making a "zzz" sound uses the more closed, adducted position of the vocal cords. This is not a bulletproof test for dysfunction, but a quick way to assess the vocal cords. Ideally you should be able to hold an "sss" sound as long as a "zzz" sound, with a ratio of 1. Dividing the time that you can sustain an "sss" sound by the time that you can sustain a "zzz" sound will give you your S/Z ratio. A ratio greater than 1.4 is considered positive for a vocal cord problem.[9] This can be used as an informal test to see if patients are able to open and close their vocal cords and, indirectly, as a way to assess the range of motion and coordination of the vocal cords. Also, comparing attempts prior to therapy with later attempts is a quick way to evaluate progress.

Use Your Voice to Assess Your Vocal Cord Tightness

Try to position your breath low, below your nipple line, taking tension away from your throat. Using an "ah" sound, think about letting your vocal cords remain open; try to feel for it. Try and hold your vocal cords open by moving your breath/air with your diaphragm. Inhale at the diaphragm, through your nose, effortlessly, and let the diaphragm drop and expand all around your body. Then exhale while saying "ah". Hold the "ah" at a consistent pitch using your diaphragm and open your vocal cords.

You will notice that the pitch becomes higher when the vocal cords shorten/tighten/come together. Try not to let this happen, but don't push past this tightening as that is your current limitation. You have to keep good form — in this assessment that means keeping a GOOD CONSISTENT TUNE. Try to keep the voice coming from the diaphragm. When the diaphragm has lost its range and the pitch changes, this is another indication that your form has been lost and you can stop this test. This is showing you your ability to use your diaphragm to make noise and also the ability of the vocal cords to stay open and in a lengthened position. You can even start to add the transverse abdominis and pelvic floor to assist in pushing air up and out through your vocal cords.

HOW TO ACTIVATE, STRETCH, AND STRENGTHEN
THE LARYNGEAL MUSCLES AND VOCAL CORDS

- Open your mouth and hold it open for five to ten seconds. This helps to lengthen or open your vocal cords.
- Pretend to yawn while holding your tongue as far back in your mouth as possible. Yawn slowly, opening the vocal cords in a five- to ten-second timespan. This helps lengthen, stretch, and/or open your vocal cords.
- Stick your tongue out and hold it for five to ten seconds. This helps bring together your vocal cords or close your vocal cords.

- Pretend to gargle while holding your tongue as far back in your mouth as possible. Do this for five to ten seconds. This helps to bring your vocal cords together or close them.
- Dry swallow, squeezing all of your swallowing muscles. This helps with closing/shortening your vocal cords. Hold for five to ten seconds.
- Lightly push against a wall or heavy object and notice how the vocal cords come together. Hold for five to ten seconds.

HOW TO IMPROVE VOCAL POWER WITHOUT STRAINING:
STRAW EXERCISES

These exercises are for strengthening your vocal cord muscles without straining. Using a straw takes some stress off of the vocal cords, allowing them to more easily do their job. Some people call straw exercises semi-occluded vocal tract (SOVT) exercises. The mouth is partially occluded or closed with these exercises, therefore changing the vocal tract. It is easier for the vocal cords to vibrate because more pressure stays in the vocal tract and returns to the vocal cords.

During these exercises, there is pressure coming from the lungs to the vocal cords and, at the same time, back pressure from your lips returning to the vocal cords. These two opposing forces make the vocal cords feel like they are floating — they feel weightless. Offloading the weight allows the muscle to strengthen without coming to fatigue or causing inflammation. This is beneficial for both a strong muscle that needs to recover and a weak muscle that needs to be strengthened. It lightens the load, much like walking in water rather than on land lightens the load on the legs and spinal joints.

Try to find the right amount of air pressure with exhalation when doing straw exercises. The straw narrows the mouth and creates back pressure that helps with the position of the vocal cords. If you try to push too much air out too fast with exhalation, that higher pressure will cause air to leak out of your mouth. Your lips will not be able to hold a tight seal on the straw. Now you no longer have the same back pressure. Another thing to watch for is the vocal cords attempting to resist the air pressure and not open or stay open when exhaling.

Try straw exercises with many sizes of straw. The smaller the diameter of the straw, the easier on the vocal cords because the back pressure will be greater. The greater the back pressure, the more the vocal cords will feel like they are supported — buoyant. Progress from a smaller straw to a larger straw with these exercises.

Stretch or Lengthen Your Vocal Cords
with Straw Exercises

Restoring full range of motion of the vocal cords, as with any deep core muscle, is important for reaching your optimal potential. Progress your vocal strength by vocalizing your lowest pitch to highest pitch through a straw. Sing a song through a straw, progressing from a small straw to a larger one. These exercises will help lengthen your vocal cords. It is important to let no air escape from your nose or mouth. Air must go through the straw. Sing from the diaphragm, not the throat; the vocal cords have to be open.

Like the other deep core muscles, posture and alignment are important for keeping these muscles *turned on* and working to their full mobility and potential. All of the deep core muscles work together to help form the posture. It is cyclical. As noted previously, using the diaphragm helps to assist in opening the vocal cords. Make sure to focus on good posture while doing vocal cord exercises for optimal training.

MAKE IT A LIFESTYLE

- Take up singing.
- Try vocal lessons.
- Sing through a straw.
- Add vocal exercises to your daily routine.

REFERENCES

1. Gray H. *Anatomy of the Human Body*. 20th ed. Lewis WH, ed. Lea & Febiger; 1918. Accessed May 20, 2025. https://archive.org/details/anatomyofhumanbo1918gray/mode/2up

2. Titze IR. *Fascinations with the Human Voice*. National Center for Voice and Speech; 2010.

3. Paulsen F, Tillmann B. Structure, function, and insertion of the human vocal folds. In: Prasad VMN, Remacle M, eds. *Advances in Neurolaryngology*. Karger; 2020:1-9. Accessed May 29, 2025. https://karger.com/books/book/339/chapter-abstract/5523757/

Structure-Function-and-Insertion-of-the-Human

4.   Sendic G. Vocalis muscle. Kenhub. October 30, 2023. Accessed
     May 29, 2025. www.kenhub.com/en/library/anatomy/vocalis-
     muscle

5.   Sieroslawska A. Muscles of the larynx. Kenhub. October 30,
     2023. Accessed May 29, 2025. https://www.kenhub.com/en/
     library/anatomy/muscles-of-the-larynx

6.   Seikel J, Drumright D, Hudock D. Appendix D: Muscles of
     phonation. In: *Anatomy and Physiology for Speech, Langauge, and
     Hearing*. 6th ed. Plural Publishing; 2021. Accessed May 29,
     2025. https://www.r2library.com/Resource/Title/1635502799

7.   Hayama S, Honda K, Oka H, Okada M. Air trapping and
     arboreal locomotor adaptations in primates: A review of
     experiments on humans. *Zeitschrift für Morphologie und
     Anthropologie*. 2002;83:149-59.

8.   Naito A, Niimi S. The larynx during exercise. *Laryngoscope*.
     2000;110:1147-50. doi:10.1097/00005537-200007000-00015

9.   Eckel FC, Boone DR. The S/Z ratio as an indicator of laryngeal
     pathology. *Journal of Speech and Hearing Disorders*. 1981;46:
     147-9. doi:10.1044/jshd.4602.147

AFTERWORD

I hope that by reading this book you can *see* and *feel* the dynamic inner beauty of a properly firing and working deep core! I hope I save you from medical burdens and make your life full of wealth! I hope you FEEL really good! Remember to do mass practice — this is a ritual — and to always assess the deep core! Make sure your foundation is *turned on* — that's where your POWER hides, deep inside!

P.S. I hope you are turned on! And turning on others!

Jeanie Iverson Crawford

TURNED ON SERIES TO COME

Release Yourself

Bike Performance: Are You *Turned On*?

Run: Are You *Turned On*?

Swim: Are You *Turned On*?

www.ingramcontent.com/pod-product-compliance
Lightning Source LLC
Chambersburg PA
CBHW050634280326
41932CB00015B/2642